Natural Mother & Baby

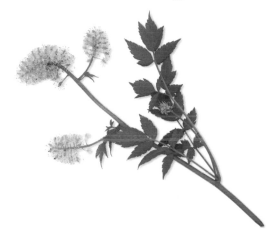

Foreword

When that little blue mark appeared on my pregnancy testing kit, the first thing I did (after sharing the monumental news with my husband) was to go and buy books on pregnancy and birth. There was naturally lots of choice but much of it seemed to focus on very technical information, the exact size of the foetus at any given month, some very scare-mongering clinical statistics and a very long list of what I mustn't eat, drink or do during pregnancy.

This book is very different, and celebrates pregnancy's holistic journey. As the introduction says 'Pregnancy is exotic and life changing'. It's so fantastic to see a book looking at the wonder of natural pregnancy and birth and within these pages you'll find a wealth of information, including excellent advice on the use of aromatherapy oils in pregnancy, beneficial therapies and treatments, and a comprehensive list of common symptoms. All against a backdrop of gorgeous pictures, and above all, a sense of great joy about being pregnant in the first place – after all, it's not a disease!

Pregnancy is often the first time many women become very conscious of putting only the most pure ingredients both into and onto their ever growing bodies. As your bump grows it's a great time to start massaging using some healing therapeutic oils and creams and what you absolutely don't need are harsh synthetic chemicals. This book outlines clearly what to avoid and indeed the wonderful natural alternatives available.

By the time I was pregnant with my 4th baby, I was so grateful to have discovered not only Neal's Yard Remedies incredible range of gorgeous natural products but also to have had the advice of their very dedicated staff's immense knowledge in this field, helping me find exactly the right products. NYR's credentials are impeccable and their organic products are not just cashing in on the 'organo-yummy-mummy' market, these are Soil Association accredited 'as pure as you can get' skincare products that don't compromise on luxury. There is a saying 'don't put anything on your skin that you can't eat' and while I may not tuck into my Organic Orange Blossom Face oil, it probably wouldn't do me any harm!

Of course food will be important to you during pregnancy and while it's important to eat healthily you'll still crave scrumptious filling food. Fear not, the recipes in here are wonderful and I'm off now to cook 'Chickpea Patties'….mmmm.
I lave a wonderful pregnancy and birth and welcome to the wonderful world of parenthood.

Janey Lee Grace is the author of Imperfectly Natural Baby and Toddler and Imperfectly Natural Home. She runs a thriving parenting forum at www.imperfectlynatural.com

Published in the UK by Neal's Yard Press
16 Stambourne Way
West Wickham
Kent BR4 9NF
e-mail: nmab@winterpress.net

NEAL'S
YARD
PRESS

ISBN 9781905830817

Printed by Biddles Ltd in the UK

Our thanks to Bridgewater for their excellent
design and to the staff and friends of Neal's Yard
Remedies for their photographs and enthusiasm.

This book is presented as a collection of natural
remedies and as an aid in understanding
their preparation and use. The book does not
represent an endorsement or guarantee as to the
efficacy of any remedy, or its preparation. The
remedies are not intended in any way to replace
or supersede medical consultation or treatment.

Contents

Introduction

Trust Your Instinct

A natural mother – deep down, every woman who has a child hopes that this is what she will be. We all want to be able to bond easily with our babies, and to understand – and meet – their earliest needs. But just as strong as this natural desire is the natural fear that we will not meet the high standards we set for ourselves. Although you may find it difficult, try to see any anxiety you feel as a reminder that you are keen to do your best, rather than a sign that you are not succeeding. And, remember, you are not the first to feel this way – and you won't be the last, either.

 Few are the mothers who have not occasionally wondered: 'Am I doing it right?'; 'Surely I could do better?'; or – when looking at other new mothers – 'Why does it look so much easier for them?' Of course, if you could get inside these other mothers' heads, you would be sure to learn that they shared all the same doubts as you. And if you step outside your own head, maybe watching yourself on a video as you go about your maternal duties – calming, cleaning and talking to your baby – you will see that, without the inner monologue that you normally run in the background, you too look like the perfect 'natural mother'.

Whether you are expecting your first child or your fourth, the first thing you need to remember is that every pregnancy, every mother and every baby is unique. No other person in the world is exactly the same as you, and you will only have this particular pregnancy once. Consider it a one-way journey to somewhere exotic and life-changing – even if you make the same trip several times, each time you repeat it your experience will be slightly different.

This is a message worth carrying with you during your pregnancy, because one thing is for sure, you will meet a lot of people – and many of them health professionals – who will try to treat you as part of a group tour, rather than an independent traveller.

A little – or even a big – part of you may be happy to fit into that group and be herded along with other new or expectant mothers: it feels safe and reassuring to

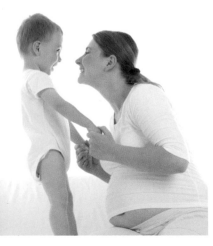

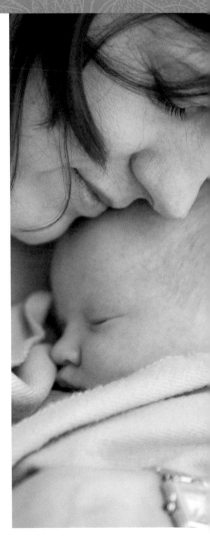

know you're not alone. Shared experiences will provide you with a wealth of essential information and support. But, even the most confident woman can be knocked off course by the sheer tide of well-meaning advice she will receive.

We have met mothers who have been highly successful in everything they have ever done – from their achievements at school to their professional and social life. Yet faced with the great unknown of pregnancy and a new baby, they are stumped. 'She should have come with an instruction manual!' they'll joke – but, inwardly they really are wishing that someone could tell them exactly what to do next. Possibly for the first time in their life, their instinct may appear to let them down.

It's not surprising – as a mother you want to do the best for your baby. But, with so much conflicting and confusing advice around, what is the best? The growth of baby manuals – especially those that are built on child-rearing schedules – is testament to the fear and anxiety that motherhood brings. We seem to have forgotten that holy grail

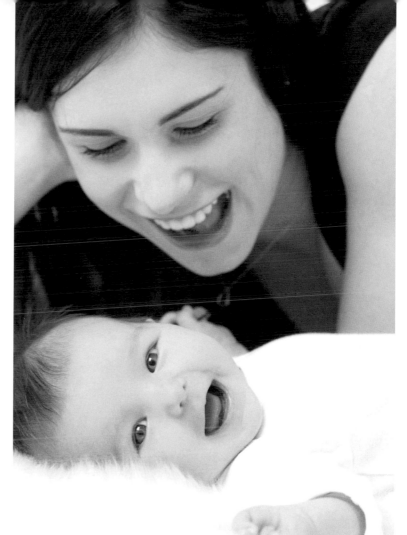

of handbooks – our own maternal instinct. This is the inner sense that tells you what is right for you and your baby. Try applying the same instinct to your neighbour's newborn and you would be quite justified in throwing your arms up and admitting, 'I'm not sure what she wants!' But deep inside you, you have a gut feeling about what your own baby wants and needs – so listen, and act on it with confidence. You're unlikely to be wrong.

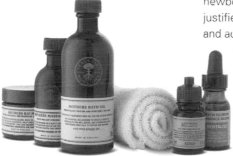

We hope this book will help you get used to listening to your instinct and acting on it – because we know how important it is to feel confident as a mother. If instinct tells you that you don't want to use chemicals on your baby, or you want to avoid medicines as far as possible, the following pages will help you find reliable alternatives. This is a book about choices and it is by exercising choice that you will become a happier, more confident, natural mother – with a baby who is also happy and secure.

Planning Ahead

Prepare Your Body

Even if you're the classic 'superwoman' – always too busy to make well-being a priority – pregnancy is one time in your life when you will want to put your health first. The general advice is for you and your partner to start looking after yourselves at least three months before you plan to conceive; but six months is even better if you want to maximise your chances of having a strong and healthy baby. This is because both egg and sperm are at their most vulnerable in the 100 days prior to conception, and you also want to ensure a healthy red cell count and a strong immune system.

You may already be in tip-top condition – taking care to eat a good range of wholesome foods, exercising regularly and avoiding alcohol and drugs. But even if this is the case, your regime is likely to need a few tweaks as you approach pregnancy.

This is a good time to find a holistic practitioner who can talk you through your body's pregnancy needs. He or she can also help you deal with any pre-existing conditions that may be worrying you. If you haven't previously been treated holistically ('as a whole person'), you will probably find the experience enlightening and

MILK THISTLE helps to cleanse the body of toxic metals

empowering. Pregnancy is often the catalyst that gets women into the habit of using complementary medicine for a whole range of conditions.

If at all possible, find yourself a therapist who is trained in a number of areas. A naturopath is a good practitioner to consult as he or she will have been trained in the way the body works and will also have an in-depth knowledge about diet, herbs and supplements that can be used to treat common problems.

Any good holistic therapist will want to take a thorough medical history from you at your first consultation, and some of the questions he or she asks may surprise you if you are only used to orthodox medicine. When you are treated holistically, everything about you is important – and the practitioner will be looking for the underlying reasons for problems, rather than the symptoms alone. If consulting a homœopath, don't be too shocked if he or she asks about your dreams and nightmares – these

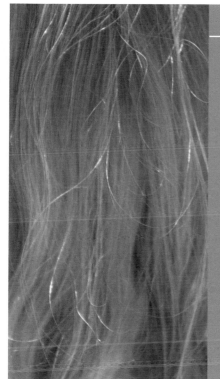

PUTTING IT ALL TOGETHER

The condition of your body now may affect your ability to get pregnant. For example, low levels of zinc have been found to prevent the fertilized egg from implanting, while zinc loss sustained in a first pregnancy can sometimes cause subsequent subfertility. To enhance your chances of a successful conception and uncomplicated pregnancy, try:

• Sticking to a diet that is organic as far as possible.
• Drinking only filtered water to avoid toxic metals, agrochemicals and excess chlorine and oestrogen.
• Hair analysis. This will reveal high levels of toxins such as cadmium and lead, which can be disastrous to foetal development, as well as mineral deficiencies – which can be equally harmful. Both can be corrected in advance of pregnancy, with the right balance of supplements and a toxin-free diet.

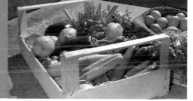

The Foresight Association for the Promotion of Pre-Conceptual Care (see page 96 for contact details) is a great source for further information.

are as relevant as the fact that you have eczema or migraines. All of this information will help the homœopath build up a picture of you as an individual (which will affect the choice of remedies for you, should you need them).

The most empowering thing about seeing a holistic therapist is that you are given the sense that you are in control of your own health, and they are there to guide you. By following the advice you're given, you will gain a deeper understanding of your body, and greater confidence in yourself as a mother-to-be.

ENJOY planning ahead for your baby's birth and parenthood with your partner

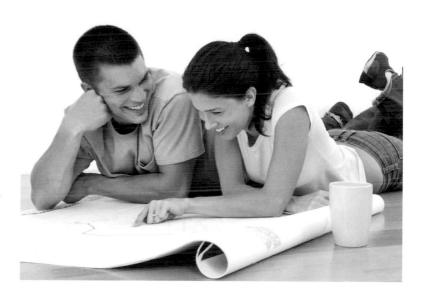

The First Trimester

Now You're Pregnant!

If you've just found out you're pregnant, congratulations! The first trimester should be a time of excitement and anticipation – even if this often manifests itself as anxiety. Remember that worrying is natural and can be seen as a sign that you're already tuning into the pregnancy. Most of the problems you encounter – like tiredness and nausea – are easily remedied and generally harmless to your baby. But a feeling that your body and life are running out of control is normal, especially when you consider the amazing changes that are taking place during this time.

 It's worth reminding yourself constantly of the enormity of your body's task during pregnancy, because then you will find it much easier to give in to the natural urge to take more rest, eat more regularly and generally let yourself be pampered. During the first 12 weeks, you are enabling a cluster of cells to develop into a foetus with a head, body, limbs, ankles, wrists, fingers and toes. By the end of the trimester this new life is even producing its own urine! And yet, as she or he is still only the size of your thumb, your pregnancy is still barely noticeable to others. In fact most women do not tell friends and work colleagues about their pregnancy until they are safely past the first trimester, because the majority of miscarriages (see box on page 11) take place during these early months.

This lack of public knowledge and acknowledgement can exacerbate feelings of anxiety and insecurity, and you may feel guilty and uncomfortable for not appearing to be your normal self, socially and at work. It helps a lot if you have a few close friends, and a supportive partner, with whom you can openly discuss all your feelings at this time – so that, privately, if not publicly, you are able to enjoy your pregnancy right from the start.

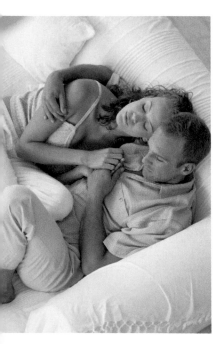

SHARING your thoughts will bring you closer as a couple

TUNING INTO YOUR PREGNANCY

Although other people may not be able to see your subtle body changes during these early months, you are likely to be very conscious of everything from your expanding waistline to your fuller breasts. You're also likely to feel overwhelmingly tired, especially in the evenings, and you may feel nauseous and notice you need to go to the loo more often. Some of these symptoms can be a pain, but the other way of looking at them is that they're your body's way of reminding and reassuring you that you are pregnant.

LOOKING AFTER YOURSELF

Letting yourself be nurtured and pampered may come easily to you – but many women find it difficult. If you're the type who normally feels guilty about indulging in a massage or facial, who eats on the go, and can't find time to exercise, then it can be hard to accept that now is a time when you need to give yourself a lot more 'me-time'. Commitments may make this seem impossible, especially if you already have other children to look after. But nurturing yourself doesn't have to be time-consuming or expensive.

Taking a few minutes here and there to relax to soft music, or to meditate (see pages 44–5), can be enormously beneficial; and making sure your diet is well balanced and that you are eating regularly is something nobody should ever feel guilty about. Exercise is important in pregnancy (see pages 30–1) but now is not the time to embark on an extreme fitness regime. It's better to sustain or build on exercise that you are already taking   walking and swimming are excellent ways to keep fit.

Three's company

Pregnancy tiredness can force you to go to bed before your partner, or to withdraw from social situations. If you do not communicate your feelings to him, not only will you be isolating yourself, but you may risk making him feel ostracised. Unless he is a mind reader, your partner may have difficulty understanding why you are acting differently these days. If you want this to be his pregnancy as well as yours, talk to him about your physical symptoms and emotions. It will help him to communicate his hopes and fears to you too.

MISCARRIAGE

One in four pregnancies ends in miscarriage, and the reasons are normally only investigated after a woman has had three consecutive miscarriages. However, Foresight (www. foresight-preconception. org.uk) can help you address nutritional or toxic imbalances that may hinder a healthy pregnancy, and the Miscarriage Association is a great source of support (www.miscarriage association.org.uk).

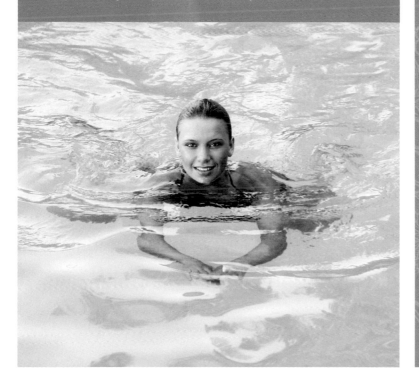

Your Pregnancy Diet

Eating For Two

Although changing your diet is always a challenge if you are set in your ways about what you like to eat, it is amazing how quickly a healthy, fresh diet can take a hold. The key is to make everything you eat as delicious as possible, using herbs and spices to maximise flavour. Processed foods are extremely addictive because of the sugar, salt and fat they contain, as well as any artificial flavourings and preservatives. They have the unfortunate effect of dulling the palate so, if you are a hardened processed food junkie, fresh and natural foods may at first taste bland in comparison.

 Once you get used to a fresh and natural diet, however, you should find that your cravings for processed food will subside and eventually vanish to the point that you have absolutely no desire to eat anything that tastes at all artificial. This is great news for your future health as well as your pregnancy. As parents, it will be crucial that you introduce your children to a varied and natural diet, and this is obviously going to be much easier if you have already established such a diet for yourselves, and built up a repertoire of simple and delicious recipes.

In animal studies, almost all commonly seen birth defects can be reproduced or eliminated by manipulating diet – removing even one essential nutrient during the crucial first trimester of pregnancy can produce the same defect across different species, and in whole litters of young. In the same animals, the situation can be reversed in subsequent litters by replacing that nutrient. Sadly, although this research has been reported in medical literature, identical birth defect tragedies continue to plague humans.

To optimise your chances of having a healthy pregnancy and baby, your diet should be broad and varied, and you should include foods from the main food groups (protein, cereals, dairy and vegetables and fruit) every day – but, in doing so, keep your diet as varied as possible and, wherever you can, eat local, seasonal and organic produce.

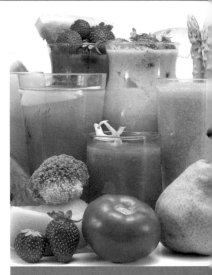

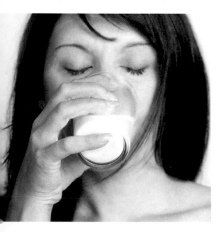

DRINKING PASTEURISED MILK is an easy way to add calcium to your diet

QUICK CHECK

- Is it fresh?
- Is it organic?
- Is it seasonal?
- Is it local?

Frozen organic vegetables are another good option, as they are frozen so soon after picking that much of their goodness is sealed in.

Wonder foods

- Sweet potato – for beta-carotene (the plant form of vitamin A) and vitamin C. Sweet potatoes are a low glycaemic index (GI) food, which means they are better for sustained energy release than white potatoes, which are high GI.
- Bananas – for a fast energy fix (they are a high GI food, but a nutritious one that should be included) and to help relieve constipation (but take care – unripe ones may cause it).
- Spinach – for calcium, magnesium, beta-carotene and iron (although meat is a better source).
- Pumpkin and squash – for fibre and beta-carotene.
- Avocados – for monounsaturated fats, fibre, vitamin E, folic acid, iron, vitamin B3 and potassium.
- Sunflower and sesame seeds – for vitamin E, omega-6 and monounsaturated fats.
- Oats – for mood-boosting B vitamins, sustained energy release and a healthy gut.
- Garlic – for healthy blood and circulation.
- Quinoa – a grain that is richer in protein than any other and also provides a range of B vitamins including B5, which strengthens the adrenal glands to help you cope with stress.
- Lentils and beans – to lower cholesterol and blood sugar levels.

Foods to eat

- Cereals – 100% whole grain flour, bread, pasta, muesli, porridge and brown rice. Include rye, barley, oats, millet, buckwheat, sesame, sunflower seeds and nuts. Buy organic to ensure that your grains are not contaminated with toxic residues from fertilisers and pesticides. Soaking grains before you eat them makes them more digestible (by breaking down complex starches such as phytates) and helps with the absorption of essential minerals.
- Dairy products – unless you are lactose intolerant (in which case, use a milk substitute made from rice, oats, nuts or soya) or have allergies exacerbated by cow's milk (in this case, goat or sheep products may be easier for you to tolerate). Make sure dairy produce is pasteurised.
- Vegetables, fruit and juices – preferably raw or very lightly cooked to preserve nutrients. Potatoes and pulses should, of course, be very well cooked.
- Protein foods – meat, poultry, game, fish, shellfish, eggs, dairy, pulses, seeds and nuts. Eat organic meat to avoid the risk of hormones, antibiotics, growth enhancers and Genetically Modified Organisms (GMOs).

ADD EXTRA VEGETABLES to a simple pasta dish for improved flavour and nutrition

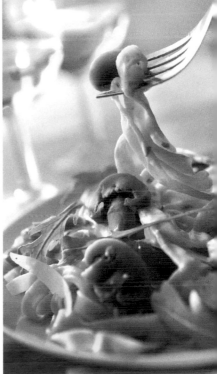

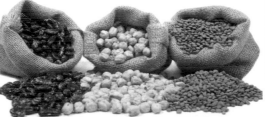

DRIED FRUITS AND PULSES are a good option for snacks and for adding protein to a meal

Foods to avoid

SUGARY SWEETS have little nutritional value and can worsen mood swings

We have just emphasised the importance of including a wide range of foods in your diet, from all four major food groups. However, there are some notable exceptions to this – foods that must be avoided or limited in pregnancy, and whose inclusion could be dangerous.

You should avoid a diet rich in processed food as it will dull your appetite for natural, whole foods, while also loading you up with sugars, which will exacerbate pregnancy mood swings and also encourage unnecessary weight gain. Also avoid salt (which can lead to high blood pressure and/or fluid retention), and saturated fat (bad for your weight and your heart). An organic diet is best as fertilisers,

lead, cadmium and antibiotics all find their way into many of the non-organic foods we buy – and in pregnancy you have two people to consider when you consume them. Food additives (sweeteners, colourings and flavourings) are also hazardous. One study found that tartrazine lowers levels of zinc in the body, by increasing urinary excretion. It has also been shown to affect the brain function and zinc status of school-age children, so it's natural to assume that unborn children would be affected too.

But even if the odd additive passes your lips during pregnancy, there are certain foods that really must be avoided at all costs.

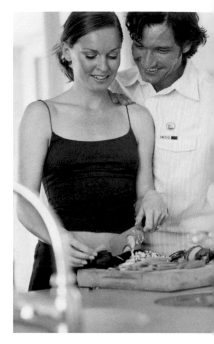

MAKING DIETARY CHANGES together will help you stick to a healthy diet

AS GOOD AS IT LOOKS?

Foods that have been grown in soil enriched with fertilisers, sprayed with organophosphate pesticides, or washed in fluoride may inhibit the use of some vital nutrient, or remove it from the body. So do make an effort to eat organic whenever possible!

Eating safely

FISH
Fish is a great source of protein and it's good to eat at least two servings a week (including one of oily fish such as fresh tuna, mackerel, salmon, sardines, trout and kipper). However, avoid shark, swordfish and marlin – these contain high levels of pollutants such as mercury, which can harm your baby's nervous system.

SUSHI
Sushi is fine to eat as long as any raw fish in it has been frozen beforehand (and it does not include the banned fish above). This may sound strange, but raw fish can sometimes contain tiny worms that could make you ill, and the freezing process kills these.

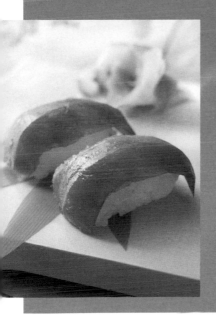

UNPASTEURISED MILK
Unpasteurised milk and cheese can contain the bacteria listeria, which, although causing only flu-like symptoms in an adult, can lead to miscarriage in early pregnancy or premature labour and the risk of stillbirth mid-pregnancy. Also avoid the soft mould-ripened cheeses such as Brie, Camembert and goat's cheese (Chèvre), along with blue-veined cheeses like Danish Blue and Stilton.

BAGGED SALADS
Bagged salads should be washed after opening, including those that come 'ready to serve', even if they have been washed in spring water. They may carry the same toxoplasma parasite that is found in cat litter, which can cause miscarriage and birth defects including brain damage. They may also carry listeria or salmonella.

PEANUTS
Peanuts are the only nut to be avoided in pregnancy – they may increase your baby's chance of developing a nut allergy, especially if anyone within the family has an allergic condition such as hay fever, eczema or asthma, which adds to your baby's risk.

UNDERCOOKED MEAT
Undercooked meat is another possible host of toxoplasma, so make sure it is cooked right through. Any wish to follow the fashion for pink beef and lamb must be put to one side for the next few months.

RUNNY EGG
Runny egg yolk runs the risk of carrying the salmonella bug, and should be avoided 'just in case'. Salmonella can cause serious vomiting, diarrhoea, fever and dehydration, and although it's most unlikely your baby will be harmed, it's best to avoid the risk. Cooking kills salmonella, so make sure you cook an egg until it is solid. For a boiled egg, that's about seven minutes. Fried eggs should be fried on both sides, and, if you're poaching, do so for five minutes. Mayonnaise – unless the shop-bought unrefrigerated variety, which is usually pasteurised and therefore safe – is made using raw eggs, and should be avoided.

LIVER
Liver and liver products such as pâté should be avoided while you're pregnant as they contain very high levels of vitamin A, which has been shown to cause birth defects. Pâté can also be a carrier of listeria.

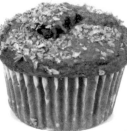

BAKE healthy wholemeal muffins for a good between-meal snack

Love your food

You have only 40 weeks of meals and snacks with which to give your baby the best possible start in life – so make sure every one of them counts. Make every bite and every calorie as healthy as you can by asking yourself: 'Will this be good for my baby?' If it's a natural, whole food, packed with minerals and vitamins, eat it. If it's packed with 'empty' calories – sweets, biscuits, crisps etc – look for something else. Don't go hungry, and, if you're really not hungry, remember your baby needs regular meals – so never skip one.

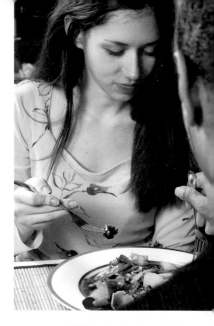

EAT A VARIETY of different coloured vegetables to help ensure you are getting the vitamins and nutrients you need

If you feel too bloated or uncomfortable with heartburn to eat normal-size meals, have six small meals spread over the day, instead of three large ones. Make a list of healthy meals and snacks you can fall back on – and, if you're a serial snacker, and have the time to bake, turn yourself into a 'cereal' snacker with home-made, low GI whole grain cakes (e.g. carrot muffins, see page 20).

In a typical day, try to include the following:

BREAKFAST
• porridge, granola or muesli with berries (see pages 20–1); or
• well-cooked eggs on whole grain toast with grilled tomatoes and mushrooms; or
• fresh fruit salad, yogurt and whole grain toast.

LUNCH
• home-made soup (see page 18) and an organic whole grain bread sandwich with tuna (once a week only), poached salmon, cheese, chicken or home-made hummus (see page 18); or

SESAME SEEDS are packed with essential fatty acids

• salad (with avocado, peppers, watercress, spinach, tomatoes, olives and onions) with brown rice, and cold chicken, fish or tofu; or
• omelette with salad and whole grain bread.

DINNER
• meat or fish and lightly steamed or stir-fried vegetables served with baked sweet potatoes, quinoa, couscous, wholemeal pasta or brown rice; or
• chickpea patties (see page 18) with salad; or
• lentils with spinach (see page 19) and grilled or pan-fried fish or tofu.

SNACKS
• nuts and seeds (though peanuts should be avoided, see page 15), fresh fruit, smoothies, yogurt or carrot muffins (see page 20).

TAKING SUPPLEMENTS

We now know about the importance of folic acid supplements in pregnancy, and of course all pregnant women are tested for anaemia in case they need iron supplements. However, while a good and wholesome diet is the cornerstone of a healthy pregnancy, there is a growing awareness that supplementation with a broad range of vitamins, minerals and fatty acids may be more important than we have previously believed. During pregnancy, larger amounts of nutrients are needed for growth and metabolism of both

your tissues and your foetus's. Even the healthiest diet will benefit from supplements. Take a specialist pregnancy supplement such as Viridian Pregnancy Complex, which contains calcium, magnesium, vitamin C, essential amino acids, potassium, docosahexaenoic acid (DHA – an omega-3 fatty acid), iron, zinc, B complex vitamins, folic acid, vitamin B6, choline, inositol, biotin, silica, beta-carotene, manganese, copper, boron, iodine,

selenium, molybdenum, chromium, vitamin K and vitamin D.

Additionally, we recommend taking a quality omega oil, such as Viridian Pregnancy Omega Oil with DHA, which is specially formulated for use during pregnancy and breastfeeding (and can help to prevent stretch marks, pre-eclampsia and post-natal depression). It contains organic golden flax seed oil, organic hemp seed oil, rice bran oil, organic avocado oil, cranberry seed oil and DHA.

VEGETARIAN OR VEGAN?

If you are vegetarian or vegan, try mixing pulses, such as chickpeas, with grains, like rice or wholemeal bread, to maximise their nutritional value. The Vegan Society (www.vegansociety. com) and the Vegetarian Society (www.vegsoc.org) are great sources of information and inspiration.

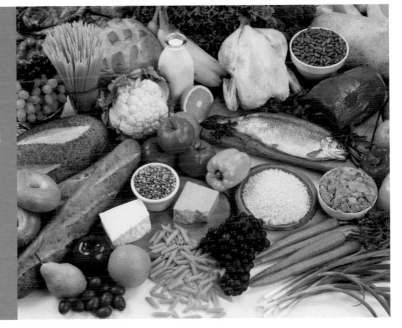

Healthy recipes

CHICKPEA PATTIES

Finely chop and sauté 1 red pepper, 1 green pepper, 1 onion and 1 clove of garlic. Season to your own taste with cumin and coriander, and add this mixture to 3 x 410 g cans of drained organic chickpeas. Blend the chickpea and pepper/onion mix in a food processor until it looks like finely ground nuts. Add chopped fresh coriander (again, according to taste), and bind the mixture with fresh lemon juice and a little yogurt until you have a dough that's moist enough to form into hamburger-sized patties. Fry these in a non-stick pan, with minimal oil, until they are brown on both sides (it takes just a few minutes) and serve with or without wholemeal buns, with salad and plain yogurt. Makes about 8 patties, and serves 4 (without buns) to 8 (with buns).

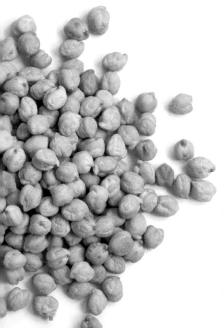

DRY CHICKPEAS should be soaked for at least eight hours and then cooked well before eating

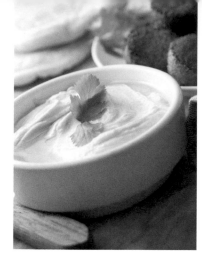

HUMMUS is delicious and very easy to make at home

HUMMUS

Drain 1 can of organic chickpeas, and whiz it up in a food processor with lemon juice, tahini, garlic, olive oil and cumin (to suit your taste). Adjust the oil, trickling it in until it reaches the right consistency for you. If it is very thick, thin it with a trickle of filtered water.

CANNELLINI BEAN AND PARSLEY SOUP

Sauté together 1 finely chopped onion, 1 carrot and 1 stick of celery in 1 tbsp olive oil. When they are softening, add 4 cloves of finely chopped or crushed garlic and soften these too. Add 2 x 410 g cans of cannellini beans, with 1.5 litres of chicken or vegetable stock. Cook together for about 20 minutes and then purée the mixture in a food processor. Return to the pan to reheat the soup, check the seasoning and add a bunch of parsley, finely chopped, and a squeeze of lemon juice. Serves 4.

SWEET POTATO, CORIANDER AND COCONUT SOUP

In a large saucepan, slowly sweat (in a little olive oil) 1 onion with 2 carrots and 2 sticks of celery, all finely chopped. When they are caramelising, add 2 finely chopped cloves of garlic and 1 tbsp each of cumin and coriander. Continue to cook on a low heat for 2 minutes, then add 4 peeled and diced sweet potatoes, with 2 litres of chicken or vegetable stock. Raise the heat and bring to a slow boil, cooking the sweet potatoes until they are soft and mushy. Now transfer the soup (in batches) to a food processor, add a bunch of washed, fresh coriander, and blend until it is a smooth consistency and the coriander is reduced to green specks. Return it to the saucepan and stir in 1 x 400 ml can of coconut milk. Serves 6.

CORIANDER adds frangrance to home-made soup

PUY LENTILS WITH SPINACH

This is a great dish to serve with grilled or pan-fried fish, or tofu, but it's also delicious on its own – and nutritious, served with brown rice or whole grain bread.

Cook 250 g of Puy lentils in plenty of water until they are tender – this takes 20–30 minutes from the time the water comes to the boil, at which point reduce the heat to a simmer. Drain the lentils and put them into a large sauté pan with 1 tbsp of olive oil and the juice of a lemon. Stir in one bag of freshly washed spinach leaves until they wilt. Now you have a choice: you can make the dish creamy, by stirring in a few spoonfuls of crème fraiche or a small pot of

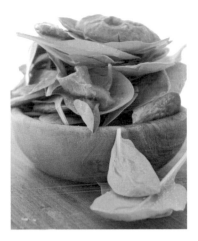

plain yogurt; or it is also very nice mixed with home-made tomato sauce (most simply made with 1 x 400 g can of organic chopped tomatoes, 1 crushed garlic clove and a large splash of olive oil, simmered together for about 20 minutes).

PUY LENTILS add substance to any dish

BABY SPINACH leaves are great in salads too

QUICK CHECK

- Am I eating regularly?
- Am I making every calorie count?
- Is my diet varied?
- Am I including every food group, and getting a good range of foods from each?
- Am I managing to avoid 'empty' calories like sugars, saturated fats and processed white flour?

SWEET POTATOES

The sweetness of sweet potatoes comes from easily digestible sugars. This makes them a good source of energy which is tempered by the high fibre content. Try baking them in their jackets, or using them in both sweet and savoury dishes.

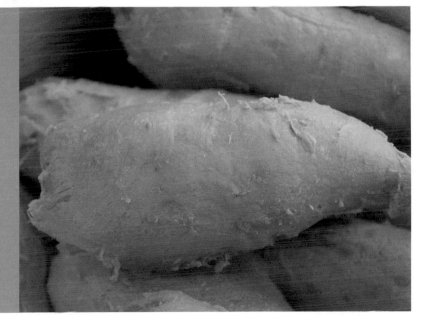

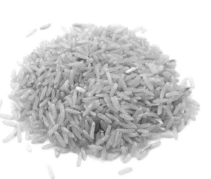

BROWN RICE is a tasty, low GI food

AROMATIC BROWN RICE
Fry a finely chopped onion in vegetable oil. Stir in your measured quantity of brown basmati rice, along with two and a half times as much water, with spices of your choice such as cardomoms, cloves, cinnamon, cumin or garam masala. Bring it to the boil, turn down the heat and simmer for 40 minutes.

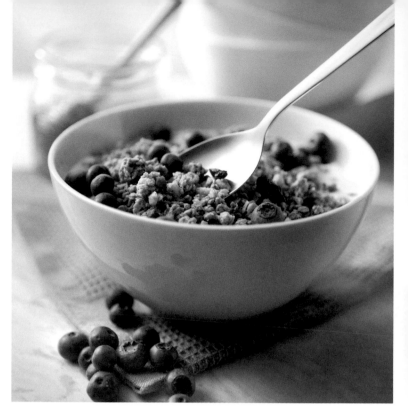

A BOWL OF GRANOLA and fresh fruit can pack goodness into your breakfast

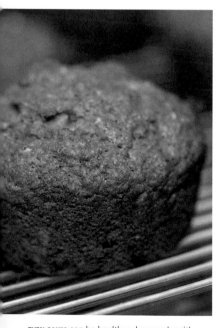

EVEN CAKES can be healthy when made with low GI ingredients

SPICY CARROT, NUT AND RAISIN MUFFINS
Preheat the oven to 190°C, gas 5. Combine your dry ingredients in a bowl: 125 g wholemeal flour with 20 g wheat bran, 40 g ground flaxseed, 2 tbsp sugar, 2 tbsp xylitol, 2 tbsp baking powder, ½ tsp bicarbonate soda, 1 tsp ground cinnamon, 1 tsp nutmeg and 1 tsp ground ginger. In a separate bowl, whisk 2 medium free-range eggs with 284 ml buttermilk and 4 tbsp vegetable oil. Stir in 1 large finely grated carrot, 75 g raisins (softened in hot water and drained) and 40 g chopped pecan nuts. Fold in the dry ingredients and pour the batter into small paper cases. Bake for 20–25 minutes until they're firm to touch. Makes about 12.

CRUNCHY GRANOLA
Preheat the over to 160°C or gas 3. Line a large shallow baking dish with greaseproof paper. Combine 500 g rolled oats with 2 tbsp each of sunflower seeds, pumpkin seeds, almonds, hazelnuts, and pecans. Mix the dry ingredients with 8 tbsp of honey and 8 tbsp coconut butter, which you've gently heated in a small pan. Spread this mixture over the prepared dish and bake for 25 minutes, stirring it halfway through cooking. As soon as you take it out of the oven, toss in dried fruit of your choice, such as raisins or chopped apricots. Leave the granola to cool completely and then store it in an airtight container. Enjoy as a snack on its own, or add milk and fresh fruit for a healthy meal.

HOME-MADE MUESLI

For one serving, soak 4 tbsp rolled oats with 2 tbsp oat germ overnight in 100 ml skimmed milk. Just before serving, stir in a little orange juice with some grated apple, and nuts and berries of your choice, and serve it with yogurt and honey.

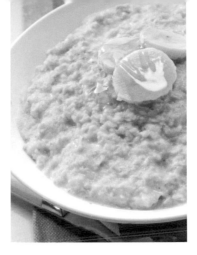

PORRIDGE made with skimmed milk helps lower cholesterol levels

FRUIT AND SPICE PORRIDGE

Cook the porridge oats in milk, water, or a mixture of both according to your taste. When it starts to thicken up, add chopped fresh and dried fruit – grated apple, chopped dates and sliced banana work well. When it's ready to serve, stir in a pinch of cinnamon, and sprinkle seeds and chopped nuts on the top. Sweeten with maple syrup or honey to taste, or a short-cut compote of raspberries or blueberries, made by putting the frozen fruit in the microwave and cooking for 1 minute.

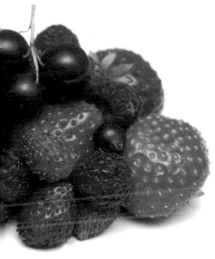

FRESH BERRIES are an easy way to add natural sweetness and nutrition to a meal or snack

SEED AND NUT SNACK

Toss together a few handfuls each of cashew nuts, pine kernels, pumpkin seeds, sunflower seeds, sesame seeds and linseed with soy sauce. Roast them in a pre-heated wok, shaking and stirring quickly until the mixture turns golden brown. It should take no more than a minute. Cool the mixture and store in an airtight container.

GARLIC SESAME FISH

Mix 4 tbsp sesame seeds with 1 tbsp chopped garlic, and spread out on a large plate. Take four fish fillets and press both sides of each into the seed mixture to coat them. Heat a non-stick pan and add a little sesame oil, and cook the fish for 2–3 minutes on each side. Serve with lemon wedges, and stir-fried spinach.

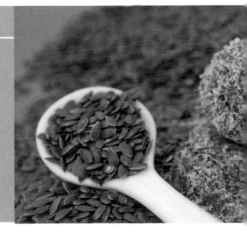

MACKEREL is an excellent source of omega 3 fatty acids, selenium and vitamin B12

EXPERIMENT WITH SEEDS

Hemp seeds and linseeds (flax seeds) may look like bird food to you, but they're the richest source of omega-6 and omega-3 essential fatty acids – both needed for brain and nerve cells, and pretty much all of our body functions.

The supreme nutritional benefits of hemp seed is that its oil provides a perfect ratio of omega-6 and omega-3 fatty acids. Along with other seeds, hemp and linseed also contain zinc, calcium and magnesium.

First Trimester Issues

Understanding Your Symptoms

Whether it is increased fatigue, nausea, or an aversion to certain foods and cravings for others, your body is sure to find ways to keep on reminding you that you're pregnant. Most women have at least one of these symptoms of pregnancy, and those who do not feel any different to usual can find it quite disconcerting. So embrace those symptoms happily – and know that, for most, there are simple, natural solutions.

 In the first trimester, typical problems are likely to include the following:

Needing to urinate more often

In the first trimester this is caused by the greater volume of body fluids you are producing: your kidneys are responding by speeding up the process by which they get rid of the waste products. As your uterus grows, the extra pressure it puts on your bladder will exacerbate the situation, but this should ease a bit after the fourth month when the uterus rises into the abdominal cavity. In the meantime, try to lean forward when you urinate to make sure you empty your bladder fully; and, to avoid too many trips to the loo at night, try not to drink a lot in the last two hours before bed.

Acupuncture, craniosacral work and osteopathy can all help a lot if the problem becomes a nuisance.

Nausea/morning sickness

Over 80 per cent of pregnant women suffer with some level of morning sickness, thought to be caused by chemical by-products of increased hormonal activity building up and creating general toxicity in the body. Get as much rest as you can and take your time getting up in the morning. Go for gentle walks – the fresh air and exercise will help (and, according to Ayurvedic practitioners, walking in fresh air will reduce the unresolved anger or 'pitta'-type stress that manifests itself as nausea in pregnancy). If the

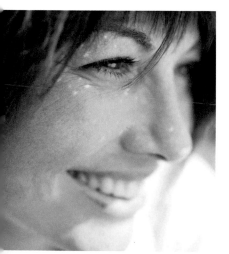

FRESH AIR can help to reduce your nausea

LISTEN TO
YOUR BODY

Taking plenty of
rest eases morning
sickness and helps you
cope with the tiredness
that can overwhelm
you in pregnancy.

problem is at all severe, then you must talk to your doctor or midwife about it.

The acupressure points for nausea are at the base of the wrist so acupressure wristbands sold for travel sickness can work very well for morning sickness, while visiting an acupuncturist can help with more severe nausea. Another great remedy for morning sickness is a slice of fresh ginger – just add to a cupful of hot water and sip as a spicy tea.

Homœopathy can also be really effective as a safe way of relieving morning sickness – choose from the following:
• Ipecac 30c (one or two doses a day) for persistent nausea that is not relieved by vomiting.
• Pulsatilla 30c (one or two doses a day) for nausea without much vomiting that is greatly relieved in fresh air – especially if you are feeling more weepy and emotional than usual.
• Sepia 30c (one or two doses a day) for nausea that is greatly aggravated by the thought or smell of food, even though it may be relieved by eating. You may experience a weak, sinking sensation in the stomach.

Tiredness

Your body is working hard all the time during pregnancy, even when you're resting, so it's little wonder you're so tired. See pages 26–7 for sleeping tips, and be careful not to overdo anything – your body is telling you it needs time off. Evening primrose oil can help

FIND THE ACUPOINT for nausea on the inside of your wrist

counter the effects of tiredness. Drink mild herbal teas such as lemon balm or chamomile instead of drinks containing caffeine, as this will make the slump in energy worse after a while.

Cravings

Although common in pregnancy, cravings for the wrong types of food (sweets and ice cream) are less likely if you stick to your healthy diet and avoid too much sugar and fat. Make sure you have a really nutritious diet, full of vital, organic foods.

Food aversions

Although it's good to go off foods that are bad for you in pregnancy (e.g. coffee

MARIGOLD has useful antiseptic and healing properties

and alcohol) – and many women do – an aversion to a healthy food can be a problem, and may be a sign of zinc deficiency, so check that your diet includes enough zinc-rich foods, such as meat, nuts, oats, potatoes and shellfish.

Bleeding gums

Raised levels of the hormone progesterone softens gums and increases blood flow, and this can result in bleeding gums. Visit your dentist, and use diluted lemon juice as a mouthwash, or combine tincture of marigold (which is antiseptic and healing) with astringent tincture of myrrh. Use the marigold and myrrh combination in a ratio of 1 part tinctures to 8 parts warm water, and swill it around in your mouth twice a day before spitting it out.

Spotty skin

If, instead of a glowing complexion, you're plagued with acne in pregnancy, there are several natural remedies that can help. The homœopathic remedy Kali ars 6c can be taken twice a day for two to three weeks, while nettle and dandelion teas help to clear the toxins that result in spots. Echinacea is also safe to take in pregnancy and will help to avoid the spots becoming infected. You can also dab neat hypericum and calendula tincture (hyper/cal) on the spots, or try Mahonia Clear Skin Gel made by Neal's Yard Remedies.

Tender breasts

It's not unusual for breasts to be agonisingly tender in the first trimester. Wear a well-fitted bra and soothe your breasts with compresses of lavender or damask rose flower water.

EATING LINSEEDS can help to relieve constipation

Constipation

Sluggish elimination is due to the muscles around your bowel beginning to relax – but don't ignore the problem as it can lead to haemorrhoids. Keep your diet rich in fruit and vegetables, and drink plenty of water. Try soaking prunes in water or cold tea overnight to eat with live yogurt for breakfast or add a tablespoonful of linseeds to muesli or porridge. Massaging your tummy in a clockwise direction, starting at the left, can help to move things along too. An acupuncturist can restore natural contractions of the colon by working on the large intestine and liver meridians. At home, gently apply acupressure to the point three finger widths below your navel.

Headaches

Pregnancy headaches are often caused by hormonal changes, but can also be due to tiredness, stress and hunger – so, as ever, make sure you get plenty of rest and eat regularly. Massaging one drop of lavender essential oil into the temples may help. Meditation, visualization and neck exercises are also very useful. If you get a migraine, try the reflexology trick of squeezing the tips of your big toes; or press on the acupoint liver 2 (on the top of the foot in the web between the big and second toes) for two minutes.

LAVENDER helps to ease headaches

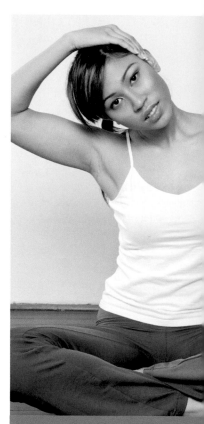

TRY YOGA

Yoga really isn't all about getting into awkward postures. There are plenty of gentle stretches, such as placing your hand on the side of your head and gently applying pressure to bring your ear towards your shoulder, which will help to release any tension in your neck that can lead to a headache.

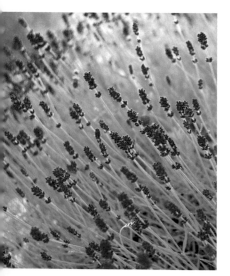

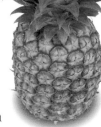

PINEAPPLE and papaya assist digestion

Heartburn

Heartburn is caused by the relaxation of the ring of muscle separating the oesophagus from the stomach, which leads to harsh digestive juices travelling back up to the oesophagus. It's more likely in pregnancy because there is increased pressure on the stomach, but it can help to eat small, frequent meals rather than big, irregular ones. Chew your food thoroughly and avoid drinking or eating too many acid-forming substances – tea, coffee, spicy foods, sugar, cakes, biscuits and so on. Papaya and pineapple both aid digestion, so try to eat them at some point during the day if you are prone to heartburn; or chew two to four papaya enzyme or pineapple bromelain tablets with a meal. Sipping chamomile or lemon balm tea can be very helpful or you could try taking the homœopathic tissue salt Nat phos 6c three times a day to relieve symptoms of acidity and indigestion.

Dizziness and fainting

While fainting itself is actually rare (and won't harm your baby), dizziness is common in the first trimester and is due to the

CAUTION!

It is best to avoid taking any medication in pregnancy that is not vital to maintaining your health, and herbal remedies should also be treated with caution. If in doubt, check with a medical herbalist before self-prescribing.

The herbs that should be avoided in therapeutic doses (unless on the advice of a medical herbalist) include aloes, angelica, barberry, bethroot, black cohosh, bloodroot, buckthorn, cascara sagrada, catnip, celery seed, cinchona, coltsfoot, cottonroot, elecampane, false unicorn, fenugreek, feverfew, ginseng, gotu kola, goldenseal, greater celandine, holy thistle, hops, horsetail, hyssop, juniper, lady's mantle, liferoot, liquorice, male fern, mandrake, marigold, milk thistle, mint, motherwort, myrrh, pennyroyal, peppermint, poke root, prickly ash, red clover, rhubarb, rosemary, rue, saffron, sage, senna, shepherd's purse, southernwood, tansy, thuja, uva-ursi, vervain, white horehound, wild indigo, wild yam, wormwood, yarrow and yellow dock.

Various essential oils should also be avoided in pregnancy – these are discussed on pages 42–3.

pressure on your blood supply to meet your rapidly expanding circulatory system. Keep your blood sugar levels stable with small, frequent, high-protein meals. Sucking on crystallised ginger can help if your dizziness is related to morning sickness. Sipping lemon balm tea can help, or try inhaling lavender essential oil from a tissue. If you are feeling generally weak and tired as well as faint from time to time, try the homœopathic remedy China 30c, twice a day for a week; or if the feelings of faintness are much worse in a warm or stuffy room, try Pulsatilla 30c.

LEMON BALM is wonderfully aromatic and can also be added to food for flavouring

How Are You Sleeping?

Fighting Insomnia

Sleep is crucial for good health at any time in your life – but especially when you're pregnant and exhausted from all the work that's quietly going on inside your body. Your normal need for eight hours' sleep a night shoots up and, ideally, you should get ten hours (eight at night and two in the day) out of every 24. Yet ironically, and very unfairly, sleeplessness is one of the symptoms of early pregnancy. If you cannot sleep for ten hours, at least try to ensure that you get as much rest as you can – in bed or on the sofa. It is much better to rest before you become completely exhausted.

 We hope you're having a good night's sleep, every night, and waking up refreshed and ready for the day. But the following are all signs that you may not be:
• You toss and turn at night, counting the hours left.
• You need an alarm to wake on time – and then snooze on in the morning.
• You use caffeine to help you stay alert in the day (definitely not recommended in pregnancy).
• You feel tired most of the time.

If you know, or suspect, you are not sleeping well, try these tips:

Have a bedtime routine

Don't do anything that will over-stimulate you in the hour before bed – no exercise (apart from sex, which can help you sleep), no TV and no work. Take a warm (but not too hot) bath just before bedtime, as raising and then lowering your body temperature will help you to feel sleepy. Adding a couple of drops of lavender essential oil diluted in a little base oil to the bath water can help to make it even more sleep-inducing.

Tune in to sleep

Use relaxing music to ease you into sleep – or a CD with a subliminal message reminding you that you are capable of sleeping well, that you will drop off easily and wake up refreshed in the morning. Tapes like these really can reach the parts your own self-talk cannot.

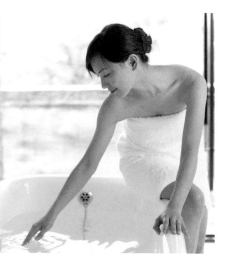

WIND DOWN with a bath before bedtime

A HELPING HAND

Your partner can help by giving you a relaxing massage before bed. Choose a blend of oils containing marjoram and lavender, as these are proven to lower levels of the stress hormone cortisol and can therefore help you both have a good night's sleep.

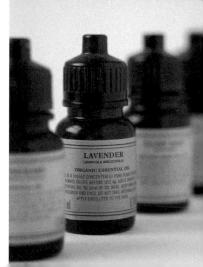

Watch what you eat

Alcohol, caffeine, cigarettes and sugary foods can all adversely affect the quality of your sleep, and are not recommended in pregnancy anyway. However, a 2005 study of people with chronic insomnia found that eating foods high in tryptophan could really help. Tryptophan raises levels of the brain chemical serotonin, which is essential for sleep. Good sources are almonds, turkey, bananas, milk, oats, wheat and eggs. One of the best sleep-inducers is a lean turkey sandwich, made with wholemeal bread and eaten mid-evening. Naturopaths associate iron deficiency with poor sleep – another reason to make sure your diet is packed with plenty of pulses, dark green, leafy vegetables and nuts if you don't eat meat.

Keep a sleep diary

Use it to log everything you can about the way you sleep – from the time you drop off and wake up, to what you eat and how you feel during waking hours. This will help you identify anything that helps or hinders your sleeping pattern.

Make your room sleep friendly

Keep it very dark and not too warm – 16–18°C (62–65°F) is ideal. Run a fan or play white noise (tuning between the channels on your radio) to drown out road and air traffic noise.

MANY HERBS are safe and beneficial in pregnancy

LAVENDER is classically calming

Sniff an essential oil

Both neroli and lavender essential oils are proven to help you sleep – add a couple of drops of either to a tissue and place on the pillow next to you.

Use herbs to relax

Gentle sedative herbs such as lime flower, passion flower, lemon balm, orange blossom, rose petal or chamomile are useful and safe to take during pregnancy. Make an infusion by adding a heaped teaspoonful of the herb or combination of herbs to a cupful of boiling water and allow to stand for 10 minutes before straining. Drink one or two cupfuls during the evening. You can add honey to sweeten the tea as this also aids sleep. A stronger sedative, valerian, should be avoided in the first trimester. If the problem is that you wake in the night and can't get back to sleep, try the homœopathic remedy Coffea 6c (especially good if thoughts racing around your mind keep you awake) or Kali phosphoricum 6c – take two or three doses hourly before bed, or a dose during the night if you wake up.

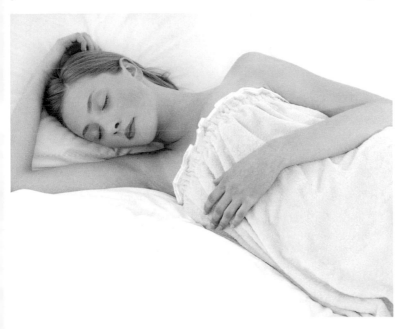

The Second Trimester

Feeling Good, Looking Great

The second trimester has a reputation for being the 'energetic phase' of pregnancy – but, remember, all things are relative! Don't expect to have more energy now than you did before you were pregnant. Although your body is usually less tired now that it has got through the strenuous first weeks of manufacturing the baby, and morning sickness may also be subsiding, a lot of your energy is still going towards nurturing your baby, who is finally making his or her presence felt in fluttery butterfly movements that will soon become unmistakable kicks and somersaults.

 You should feel your baby move for the first time around week 16 – it's called 'quickening' and feels like tiny bubbles or flutters which are so subtle at first that you have to be quite in tune with your body to notice them. It's an exciting turning point in pregnancy as, from now on, you will have a greater connection with your baby. But, ironically, the looming reality that comes with the first signs of quickening can also cause some mothers to have their first misgivings about the imminent upheaval to their lives. Don't worry about these feelings. Studies show that not only is a little ambivalence, or even fear, normal, it's also quite healthy – as long as these feelings are confronted. This is a good time to talk any worries through with your partner, and work out how you can deal with your new life as a family instead of a couple.

By the last month of this trimester – weeks 23–28 of your pregnancy – your baby is moving more vigorously and will jump at an unexpected loud noise. Sometimes he or she may get hiccups, which you may feel, and a pattern of waking and sleeping is also established – which you may also tune into, especially if he or she wakes and kicks at precisely the time you want to go to sleep. As the trimester progresses, if you have the feeling that you're missing out on your baby's movements, take a bath and gently stroke your tummy. You should be rewarded

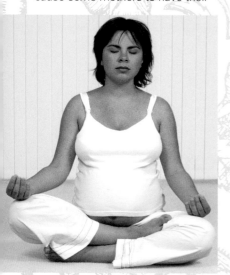

MAKE THE MOST of quiet time to tune into your body and mind

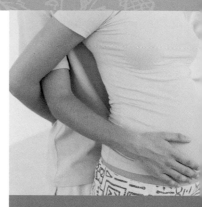

HOW MUCH WEIGHT SHOULD I GAIN?

Normal weight gain in pregnancy is 11–13 kg (24–28 lb), which includes the weight of the baby, placenta, amniotic fluid and your own body changes. If you started the pregnancy underweight, expect to gain 12–16 kg (26–35 lb). If you're overweight, expect to gain 7–10 kg (15–22 lb).

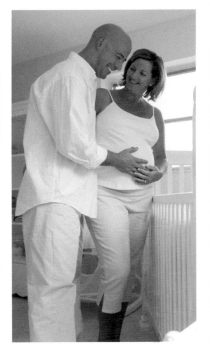

SHARING BABY KICKS with your partner can help him feel included in your pregnancy

Now's the time to...

- Book antenatal classes – they vary a lot, so do all the research you can to find one that suits you.
- Speak to your midwife about your birth plans.
- Visit the local hospital or maternity unit to see how things are done there.
- Take more exercise – swimming is excellent for your back, but don't do a version of breaststroke that keeps your head out of the water as this will put more strain on your back.
- Address your posture to prevent backache. The Alexander technique and pilates can help a great deal with this.
- Find good yoga and meditation classes that will help your body and mind relax in preparation for the latter part of your pregnancy.
- Consider rebirthing – one way of preparing yourself for childbirth using a simple breathing technique that helps liberate your body from tension, fear and pain. It can help you get in touch with your feelings so you can recognise and release any harmful memories.

with a few kicks, or an undulating stomach as the baby moves around.

As well as feeling pregnant in the sense that you are more conscious of your baby, you may suffer some of the common side effects of pregnancy, such as forgetfulness and clumsiness. Take these in your stride. Forgetting the occasional appointment and feeling as if you're losing brain cells is caused by hormonal changes. A few extra 'To Do' lists should help to minimise the disruption to your life. Clumsiness is due to a combination of factors: loosening joints, water retention and lack of concentration – all of which are an inevitable part of pregnancy. Understanding why you're more butterfingered can help you and those around you to be more patient.

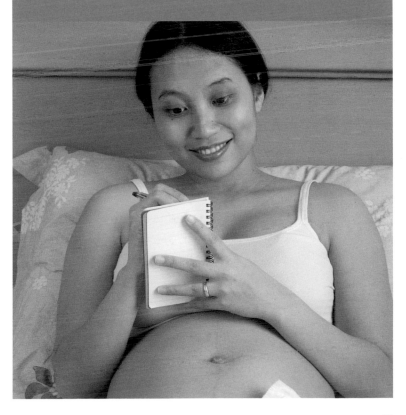

Keeping Fit

Exercising Safely

Your grandmother may have been warned not to take exercise in pregnancy, but these days it is generally considered a benefit. It helps your circulation, builds stamina for the birth and makes it easier to get back into shape afterwards. However, this is not the time to start running a marathon, and if you've been used to doing fairly strenuous sports, you must be prepared to adapt to a gentler routine. If you're not already physically active, only take up something easy such as swimming or walking – just 10–15 minutes a day is all you need to do.

 We've met women who have been happily and energetically taking part in aqua-aerobics classes right up until the day before they've given birth – but how much exercise you take depends on your level of fitness and any problems you have encountered in this or previous pregnancies. Talk to your doctor, natural health practitioner and fitness instructors about the pregnancy – their advice will be invaluable, especially if you are very fit and find it difficult to accept that you have to adapt your exercise routine.

If you already do one of the following sports, remember that pregnancy softens your joints and ligaments, making you much more susceptible to straining yourself if you overdo it.

Aerobics

Stick to a low impact class and don't jump up and down or allow yourself to become overheated. Drink plenty of water before and after classes, and limit yourself to 30 minutes.

Badminton

Overstretching and pulling muscles and ligaments is a risk, and, again, you should not jump up and down.

Cycling

As long as you don't fall off, cycling is a safe exercise, but remember that as you get bigger you will have more weight at the front, which could cause you to topple. Take it easy and go slowly – and be extra safety conscious if you're cycling down hill.

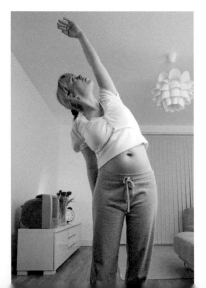

KEEP UP the good work – but don't start anything new or strenuous

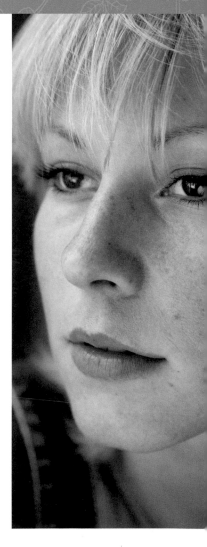

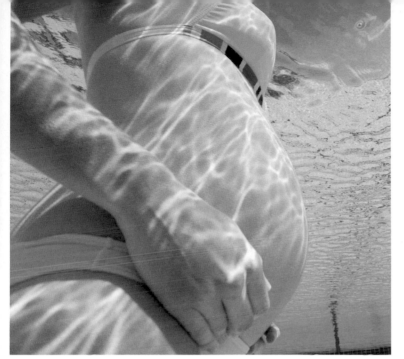

Skiing

The safest time to ski is in your second trimester – but try not to fall heavily, and avoid high speeds and crowded pistes. In late pregnancy, it becomes physically difficult, and potentially dangerous as it could induce a premature labour.

Walking

A great, low-impact aerobic exercise. If you dislike all other forms of keeping-fit, try to take a walk every day.

WATER EXERCISE provides a rare taste of weightlessness during pregnancy

Jogging

If you're already a jogger, carry on, but take some advice (from a gym instructor or physiotherapist) on adapting your stride to avoid jarring.

Water exercise

Swimming is wonderful exercise in pregnancy as your body weight is supported by the water. Just be careful not to open your legs too wide during breaststroke as this opens up the pelvis. Aqua aerobics classes are also very beneficial.

Tennis

Playing a game is OK for the first trimester, but after that stick to practising shots rather than running around on the court.

Horse riding

It's recommended that you avoid activities with the risk of hard falls, so – no matter how much of a pro you are – riding is out.

PELVIC FLOOR EXERCISES

If 'pelvic floor' sounds like something you may want to use when redecorating your kitchen, welcome to the new world of motherhood! You will now be introduced to this hitherto unnoticed part of your body for the first time.

The pelvic floor is the sling of muscles that helps hold the pelvic organs in place, and pelvic floor exercises will be important for the remainder of your life. Without them, these muscles can become slack, making sexual intercourse less enjoyable, and putting you at risk of stress incontinence. In pregnancy the increase of the hormone progesterone softens tissues, making them more stretchy. As the pelvic

floor also softens, and is under additional pressure from the weight of your growing baby, this is a good time to start strengthening it.

Lie down with your knees bent up and your feet on the floor. Tighten your vagina, urethra and anus together. Now think of the three tightened areas as a drawbridge, and try to lift it up inside you. Hold, breathing slowly in and out, then slowly let it down in as many stages as you can manage. Once you have mastered this exercise you will be able to do it anywhere – even when you are standing in a queue at the supermarket – and nobody will know!

Second Trimester Issues

What's Normal, What's Not?

Outwardly you may be blooming in the middle months of your pregnancy, but inwardly you may have worries about your future as a mother – and common pregnancy symptoms can cause you more anxiety. As with the first trimester, most are not harmful to your baby, and are a normal result of hormonal actions on the body. Use natural remedies whenever you can, but exercise common sense too, and report anything that seems abnormal to your doctor.

Abdominal pain

As the muscles and ligaments of the abdomen stretch, some degree of abdominal pain is to be expected – and this may be experienced as a sharp or crampy pain that's most noticeable when you are standing up after sitting or lying down, or when you cough. However, it's always a good idea to mention any abdominal pain to your doctor or midwife to make sure it is definitely nothing to worry about. You do need to seek urgent medical help if the pain is persistent, or accompanied by other symptoms such as fever, bleeding, vaginal discharge or faintness.

Natural remedies for the normal type of abdominal pain include drinking chamomile, lemon balm and lime blossom tea (make your own, using a heaped teaspoonful of combined herb per cup). The homœopathic tissue salt Mag phos 6c will relieve muscular aches and cramping – take one dose morning and night for a few days until the problem is relieved. For groin pain, practise yoga squats (see pages 44–5 and 51) to loosen your hips and pelvic floor.

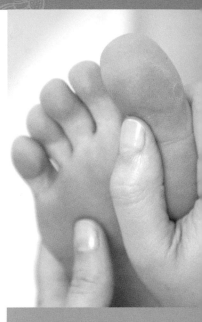

Backache

Backache is another result of your joints loosening up to prepare you for delivering your baby. Swimming is a great exercise for the back, and the yoga cat posture (see pages 44–5) is particularly good for lower back pain. A back massage with St John's Wort oil relieves pain and irritation of the nerve endings. If the pain is persistent, consult an osteopath or reflexologist.

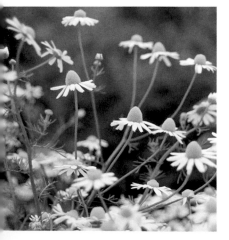

MAKE GOOD use of soothing chamomile

ACUPUNCTURE, like reflexology, can treat a range of conditions by releasing blocked energy

Blood pressure

Normal blood pressure should be 120/80. If this reading goes up to anything above 140/90 you have high blood pressure, and this is worrying in pregnancy as it can be a sign of pre-eclampsia, which is dangerous to both you and your baby. A study at St Thomas' Hospital found that a supervised course of vitamin C and E tablets in the second half of pregnancy could prevent pre-eclampsia, the theory being that your risk is greater if you have run down your essential minerals and vitamins during the course of pregnancy. Another good reason to take care of your diet!

However, not all high blood pressure in pregnancy is a sign of pre-eclampsia. Drinking lots of water, avoiding salt and taking plenty of bed rest can help bring down high blood pressure – but it's important to follow your doctor or midwife's advice about this. Garlic powder tablets have been proven to lower raised blood pressure and there's anecdotal evidence that fresh garlic combined with watercress works best – so add both to your salads!

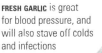

FRESH GARLIC is great for blood pressure, and will also stave off colds and infections

Hyperventilation (over-breathing) can push your blood pressure up, so learn a breathing therapy such as buteyko to slow down your breath. In studies, acupuncture has been shown to have a great effect on blood pressure; and aromatherapy, homœopathy, flotation therapy and herbalism can also help, but you will need to consult a qualified practitioner for help with this issue.

Breathlessness

Mild breathlessness is common in the second trimester, caused by hormonal actions swelling the capillaries in the respiratory tract and relaxing the muscles of the lungs and bronchial tubes, but severe breathlessness, with rapid breathing and chest pain is something you should get immediate medical advice on.

Calm mild breathlessness with frankincense oil in your bath, and practise meditation and visualisation to calm your mind if anxiety is exacerbating the problem.

Chloasma

Chloasma is a darkening of the complexion, caused by hormonal changes. The common daisy has a reputation for clearing this type of skin discolouration – make an infusion of it (2–4 g per cup of water) to dab on your skin. Foods rich in PABA (para amino benzoic acid) are also thought to help, such as wheatgerm, whole grains, mushrooms, fresh fruit and vegetables.

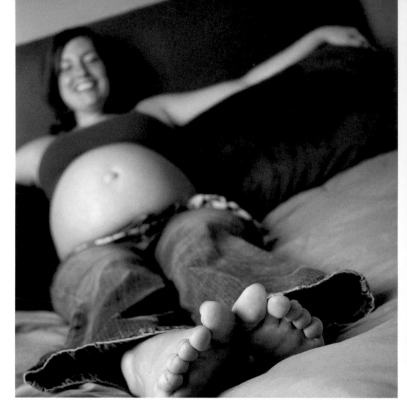

Diabetes

Diabetes is caused by a lack of the hormone insulin, which regulates blood sugar levels. The result is that sugar levels rise and this can cause problems for you and your baby. Hormonal changes in pregnancy cause blood sugar levels to go up, and most pregnant women produce extra insulin to cope with the increase. But, especially if you are overweight, this may not be effective and blood sugar levels will rise further. If you are diagnosed as diabetic in pregnancy, treatment with insulin may be unavoidable if diet alone cannot control the condition – but it is essential to be treated, as diabetes can lead to complications for your baby. Yoga can help enhance pancreatic function and improve diabetes, and Ayurvedic practitioners recommend 'bitter' foods such as green bananas. It may also be helpful to consult a qualified nutritionist or homœopath for help, but only in conjunction with advice from your doctor or midwife.

Leg cramps

Night-time leg cramps are common in the second half of pregnancy, caused by a mineral imbalance in the blood (too little calcium and too much phosphorus) – so address your diet if this happens to you. Lavender oil in your bath water or a

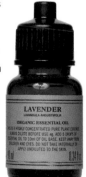

LAVENDER really is a must-have oil during pregnancy

massage from your partner (use a few drops of marjoram oil in a carrier oil) can help prevent cramps. The homœopathic tissue salt Mag phos 6c will relieve muscular cramps – take one dose as required, or take one three times a day for two weeks as a preventative measure. If you get an attack and the pain doesn't subside, get medical help.

Perineal pressure

Perineal pressure increases as the baby grows and presses down. Lie on your side to relieve the pressure, and massage the area with sweet almond oil (your partner can help), then apply a soothing pad of lavender water.

ELEVATE your feet to prevent swollen ankles

Rectal bleeding

Fresh blood from your anus is often a sign of piles (haemorrhoids), which are varicose veins in the rectum. They are common in pregnancy, and even more likely if you have been constipated. Any dark or black blood loss should be investigated by your doctor. Applying witch hazel compresses or ice packs can relieve the pain, and cypress oil can shrink piles (put a few drops in a bidet or bowl of warm water and sit in it). The herbal remedy pilewort – sold as an ointment cream – is also helpful. The homœopathic tissue salt Calc fluor 6c will help tone vein walls and help prevent piles and varicose veins – take one dose three times a day for a month.

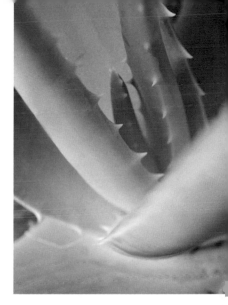

Swollen feet and ankles

Fluid retention and weight gain in pregnancy can make your feet fuller than they were before. This can also be exacerbated by the hormone relaxin, which loosens the pelvis in preparation for childbirth but also has an effect on other joints, including those in the feet. Any swelling will go down after you've had your baby, but some women will find that their joints never fully tighten up, leaving them with a bigger shoe size for life. Wear comfortable, low heeled shoes in breathable material. Take regular gentle exercise to keep the fluids and blood pumping through your circulation and also get plenty of rest with your feet elevated.

Massage your feet and ankles with a couple of drops of geranium and cypress essential oils diluted in a vegetable oil base.

Thrush

Hormonal changes in pregnancy make you 10–20 times more likely to get vaginal thrush, but the active ingredient fluconazole in oral thrush treatments is not safe to take in pregnancy, so use natural remedies. Try soaking a cotton sanitary pad in an infusion of marigold, sweet violet and golden seal (equal parts diluted one part to 15 parts of water) with one drop of tea tree oil, and wear next to your skin for two hours at a time. Aloe vera juice can be applied using cotton wool as a cooling and soothing lotion. You should also cut sugar out of your diet and eat plenty of live yogurt, or take probiotic (acidophilus) capsules. You can use a mixture of lavender, palmarosa and tea tree oils (add two drops of each to 10 ml base oil or full fat milk) in your bath.

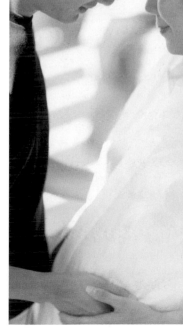

DO I NEED TO SEE A DOCTOR?

Always seek medical advice for the following symptoms:

- Vaginal bleeding
- Pain when urinating
- Severe abdominal pain
- Fluid from the vagina, which could be leakage of your amniotic waters
- Change of baby movements – especially if they diminish
- High fever or chills
- Severe vomiting
- Blurred vision
- Severely swollen face or fingers
- Severe headache

- Any injury or accident, such as a fall, which you fear could have harmed your baby
- Breast lumps
- Leg pain – especially when squeezing the calf or walking, which could be a sign of deep vein thrombosis
- Dizziness, which could be linked to high blood pressure or anaemia
- Excessive itchiness, especially of the limbs

DIY Pharmacy

Pamper Yourself

Your skin can change dramatically in pregnancy, becoming oilier or drier than usual, and sometimes swinging between extremes. You may be reluctant to use chemical-based products at this time, and it is extremely satisfying to make your our own skin-pampering products and know exactly what has gone into them – and what will go into your skin.

 The following recipes have been devised by Neal's Yard Remedies' aromatherapist Emma Thomson, and all make 100 ml. They are based on oils renowned for being both safe and beneficial to use during pregnancy. Make sure you store the oils in a dark bottle away from heat and light.

First trimester
BALANCING SKIN OIL

This blend concentrates on balancing the emotions and giving energy at a time when you can feel exhausted. Apply morning and night all over your body, and your face if you wish.
Use organic base oils and essential oils where you can.

BASE OILS
20 ml of almond oil
20 ml of grapeseed oil
20 ml of coconut oil
10 ml of jojoba oil
10 ml of apricot
  kernel oil
10 ml of avocado oil
10 ml of wheatgerm oil

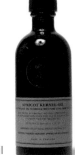

BASE OILS nourish the skin

AROMATHERAPY OILS
8 drops of neroli essential oil
5 drops of mandarin essential oil
4 drops of olibanum essential oil
3 drops of grapefruit essential oil

Second and third trimester
RELAXING SKIN BLEND

This blend will help hydrate skin and encourage sleep and relaxation at a time when sleep can become difficult to obtain.
Use the same base oils as above, but add:
1 tablespoon of calendula macerated oil
5 drops of lavender essential oil
5 drops of geranium essential oil
5 drops of olibanum essential oil
3 drops of vetiver essential oil
3 drops of bergamot essential oil

BATH TREATS
Baths are a great way to unwind throughout pregnancy.

A wonderful treat, which also deeply hydrates the skin, is Cleopatra's Linden Beauty

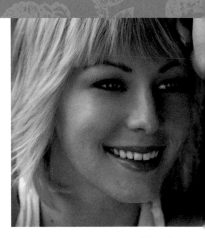

FEEL GOOD about pampering yourself by using natural products

Bath. The lactic acid in the milk is deeply relaxing and the honey and essential oils are luxurious and calming. Linden (lime) flowers have a deeply sedative effect on the mind and body – make enough tea so that you can also sip a cupful while in the bath.
You need to make this up fresh every time you use it:
• In a saucepan, heat 100 ml of full fat organic milk with 1 tsp of runny organic honey. Do not boil.
• Pour boiling water over 2 tbsp of dried lime flowers and strain after 10 minutes.

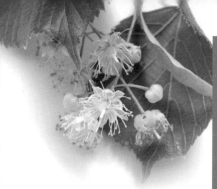

LINDEN FLOWERS are deeply calming

- Add the lime flower tea to the milk and then add 5 drops of ylang-ylang essential oil and 3 drops of vetiver essential oil
- Run your bath, pour in the mixture, sit back and relax for at least 20 minutes.

**ROSEMARY AND
MINT FOOT REVIVER**

Feet can get both tired and achy during pregnancy – the mint and rosemary are naturally cooling and invigorating.

Marbles or smooth pebbles are a lovely way to relax the feet – just sit down and run your feet over them. Putting the marbles in the fridge before use makes them extra refreshing.

- Pour boiling water over two sprigs each of fresh rosemary, mint and lemon balm and set aside to infuse for at least 10 minutes.
- Refrigerate until cool, then add 1 drop of peppermint essential oil. If you want, you can add the cold marbles or pebbles and ice cubes to really cool the legs – place everything in a large bowl and sit with your foot in it for at least 20 minutes. You can also put this mixture in a spray bottle and carry it round with you to use whenever you need it.

Mini facial routine

Not everyone looks radiant in pregnancy – sadly, for some of us, lack of sleep and hormonal changes leave our skin lacking that pregnant glow. Introducing a mini facial into your routine at least once a week will make a huge difference, and help with sleep too.

- Add 2 drops of lavender essential oil and 1 teaspoon of dried lavender flowers (optional) to a bowl of warm water, then dip a flannel in the water, squeeze out the excess water and apply to the face.
- Once the pores have opened, cleanse with a balm base cleanser (such as Neal's Yard Remedies Wild Rose Beauty Balm) for normal or drier skins, or a foaming cleanser (such as Palmarosa Facial Wash) for greasy skins. Remove with the warm flannel.
- Use a clay mask, or Neal's Yard Remedies Palmarosa Facial Mask, on greasy or problem skin. For drier skin, apply a home-made avocado and honey face pack – add a mashed ripe avocado to 5 ml of clear organic honey, 5 ml of lemon juice and 5 ml of full fat plain yogurt. Mix together and apply to the face. Remove after 10 minutes.
- Finish your mini facial routine with a facial massage using Neal's Yard Remedies Orange Flower Facial Oil, working upwards and concentrating on the cheeks and forehead. You can leave the oil on your skin overnight to penetrate the skin.

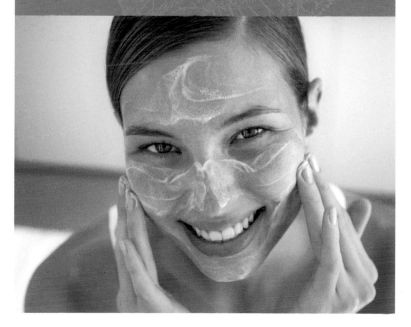

Choosing a therapy

ACUPUNCTURE

Practised in Eastern countries for 2,500 years, this is a traditional Chinese medicine based on the understanding that our body's motivating energy force, or qi (pronounced 'chi'), moves through a network of channels or meridians that run beneath the skin. Illness is caused by blockages in this flow of energy.

HOW IT WORKS
A therapist will insert fine, sterile needles at certain points along the body's meridians to restore the flow of qi.

PREGNANCY USES
Acupuncture is safe and effective to use for a range of problems from migraine and sciatica to labour pain and poor milk supply when breastfeeding. A therapist can also show you key acupoints that you can work yourself, applying gentle acupressure (without needles).

AROMATHERAPY

Plants contain a vital life force or essence that we can access through the aromatic oils they produce. The healing properties of these oils bring relief to a range of physical and emotional problems and aromatherapists are highly knowledgeable about what can be used, and when.

HOW IT WORKS
A therapist will spend time taking a full medical history before blending oils according to your personality as well as your symptoms or underlying health concern. The oils are usually applied in a relaxing massage, which enables the oil molecules to pass into the bloodstream and nervous system.

PREGNANCY USES
A growing number of midwives are now employing aromatherapy to help their patients through labour. For more information about the benefits – and the oils to avoid – see pages 42–3.

BOWEN TECHNIQUE

This is a gentle, subtle form of massage from Australia.

HOW IT WORKS
Practitioners use their thumbs and fingers to make rolling-type movements on affected areas of the body, to calm muscles, ease soft tissues and allow normal energy flow in the body.

PREGNANCY USES
Particularly good for musculoskeletal problems (such as back pain). Avoid Bowen massage around the abdomen in the first trimester.

CHIROPRACTIC/ McTIMONEY

These are related therapies that treat ill health by remedying underlying misalignments in the spine, which disrupt surrounding nerves. These misalignments may result from accidents or injuries, or from poor posture, stress and over-exhaustion.

HOW IT WORKS
Practitioners use their hands to mobilise and gently adjust the joints and muscles of your whole body to restore normal alignment.

PREGNANCY USES
Vigorous manipulation of the spine isn't recommended in pregnancy, so always tell a practitioner you are pregnant. The treatment can help post-natally, to redress misalignments caused by the pregnancy or childbirth.

CRANIAL OSTEOPATHY

Also called craniosacral therapy, this is a very subtle hands-on therapy that relieves stress and tension in the body.

HOW IT WORKS
Cranial osteopaths are trained to feel for subtle changes in the cranial rhythm of the body's tissues. Working on the skull, they improve the circulation of cerebrospinal fluid. The treatment involves touching and tapping, rather than any obvious manipulation of the skull bones.

PREGNANCY USES
This treatment may help with fertility problems, if a trauma has affected the way the bones in the head move resulting in some restriction of the pituitary gland, which controls reproductive hormones. It can also help with problems such as frequent urination; but it really comes into its own in the treatment of babies who have had assisted deliveries (for example, with forceps or ventouse). See pages 84–5.

FLOWER REMEDIES

Flower essences have numerous applications to treat emotional problems. The aim is to restore health and happiness.

HOW IT WORKS
After a full medical history, a therapist will prescribe flower essences for you to take in drops added to a glass of water.

PREGNANCY USES
Some essences are particularly good for pregnancy; mimulus treats feelings of fear (of the birth, pain or complications), while walnut is useful if you feel unsettled about the big life change ahead.

HERBAL MEDICINE

Probably one of the most commonly practised forms of medicine worldwide, but relatively new to the West, herbalism can be used alongside conventional modern medicine to treat a range of conditions. Herbal pharmacists argue that the complex mix of substances present in their herbal remedies are naturally well balanced, making them safe and effective.

HOW IT WORKS
A full medical history and examination should be taken before herbs are prescribed, and some practitioners will use complementary methods of diagnosis, such as iridology. Prescribed herbs may be given as a pill, powder or tincture, or as a tea. There's a growing number of over-the-counter herbal remedies available, but we recommend that you use only those that are either licensed herbal medicines or carry a 'traditional herbal remedy' license. From 2011, all herbal remedies will have to carry one of these licenses.

PREGNANCY USES
Herbal medicines can be very potent, so it is important to check with a therapist before self-prescribing. However, some are safe to use at home – for example, calendula (marigold) as a soothing soak for vaginal infections, psyllium for constipation, and parsley (add it to your salads) for anaemia. See page 25 for the herbs you must avoid in pregnancy.

Choosing a therapy

HOMŒOPATHY

Homœopathy is a system of complementary medicine that stimulates the natural healing mechanisms within the body so that it can heal itself.

HOW IT WORKS

The system bases itself on several natural laws of health and illness and on a set of principles for treatment. Homœopathic remedies are made from natural substances and there is a special pharmacological process that is followed to create the medicines that involves diluting the substance and then vigorously shaking it. This is thought to release the necessary traces of the substance into the carrier liquid (usually water or alcohol), thus creating a new form of the substance as a homœopathic remedy.

PREGNANCY USES

Homœopathy is a completely safe form of treatment and therefore is often used in pregnancy and childbirth, when other medicines are restricted. In fact, pregnancy is often the first exposure that many people have to homœopathy. It can provide a relief of minor symptoms throughout the pregnancy and birth, and help with breastfeeding and minor infant complaints.

NATUROPATHY

A complete health system, concerned with treating the whole person.

HOW IT WORKS

A naturopath's key role is to educate you about your health, and how to maintain it – a lot of the advice you get is based on common sense, but naturopaths are highly trained to understand how the healing mechanisms in the body work and are very knowledgeable about nutrition and herbs.

PREGNANCY USES

This is an excellent way of preparing for childbirth, as the basis of naturopathy is a healthy lifestyle. Both you and your partner could attend for a consultation and get fit together. Naturopathy is particularly good for digestive problems, tiredness, anaemia and stress.

NUTRITIONAL THERAPY

Good nutrition is vital for a healthy body, and a nutritional therapist can look closely for areas where yours can be improved. She or he can also identify food intolerances that may need to be addressed.

HOW IT WORKS

A nutritional consultation gives you the tools to nourish your body and take control of your health with various foods and supplements of herbs, minerals and vitamins.

PREGNANCY USES

Great for optimising your health and energy levels and preparing for early motherhood, when nutritional deficiencies can impact on breastfeeding, energy levels and mental health.

OSTEOPATHY

This is a system of diagnosis and treatment that corrects imbalances in the structure of the body.

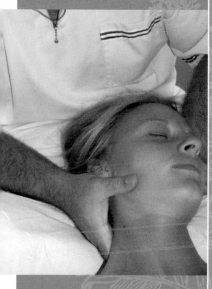

HOW IT WORKS

An osteopath will examine and palpate the spinal column, looking at your levels of mobility.

PREGNANCY USES

Osteopathy can be used for a wide range of muscular or joint problems in pregnancy, especially back pain, sciatica, neck pain and headaches – but always tell a practitioner that you are pregnant before he or she starts any manipulation.

REFLEXOLOGY

This is an ancient Eastern healing tradition based on the principle that all parts of the body are connected by energy pathways, which end in the hands, feet and head.

HOW IT WORKS

Reflexology involves a relaxing foot massage, as the therapist works through the organs and systems of the body, which are reflected in the feet. Expect to feel some pain in areas that are sensitive elsewhere in the body.

PREGNANCY USES

Very good for minor health problems (aches and pains), but comes into its own as a treatment for pain relief in labour, or for shortening a long labour by stimulating the release of oxytocin, which then helps the uterus to contract.

SHIATSU AND TUI NA

These ancient Chinese methods of massage are based on the concepts of internal energy (qi), yin and yang and the acupuncture meridians.

HOW IT WORKS

You lie comfortably on a mat, while your practitioner stimulates various acupuncture points over your body, using fingertips or hands, elbows and even feet.

PREGNANCY USES

Shiatsu can help with stress and anxiety in pregnancy, and is also useful to help you relax during labour.

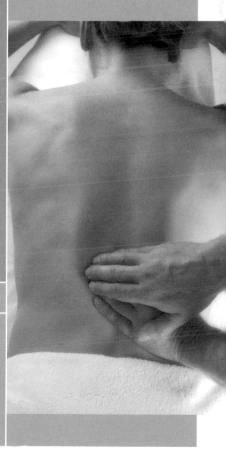

Aromatherapy in Pregnancy

Flower Power

Aromatherapy is one of the oldest forms of medicine, dating back 6,000 years to Ancient Egypt, India and Persia. Aromatic oils were brought to Europe by the Crusaders, and by the Middle Ages they were being used as perfumes and medicines. In the last 30 years, aromatherapy has enjoyed a huge revival. In France, doctors often use essential oils as an alternative to antibiotics, and the oils are often chosen by pregnant women who wish to avoid proprietary medicines. However, do remember that the oils are powerful substances, and should always be diluted properly and handled with care.

 Many studies have shown that when applied to the skin or inhaled, essential oils are absorbed into the bloodstream and metabolised by the body. In an eight-year-long study of 8,058 British women given aromatherapy during labour, 54 per cent found lavender helpful and 64 per cent benefited from frankincense. The oils have many other uses throughout pregnancy, too, with the added advantage that they are easy to use – and are a great way to involve your partner, who can help to blend the oils and massage you. But there are safety considerations to be followed:

• Firstly, essential oils should never be used internally without proper medical advice and there are a few essential oils that should be avoided altogether during pregnancy, such as basil, hyssop and sage. For best results take advice from a qualified aromatherapist (see www. aromatherapycouncil.co.uk for acceptable qualifications).

• Secondly, essential oils are extremely concentrated and need to be diluted in a suitable base oil before use. In pregnancy, a typical dilution would be 2 per cent – this translates as 10 drops of essential oil to 2 teaspoons of carrier oil. You should also only use good quality pure essential oils and pure cold pressed vegetable carrier oils such as sunflower, sweet almond or olive oils.

• Safest to use are the following oils: geranium, mandarin, neroli,

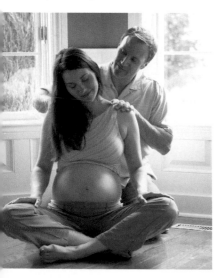

ENJOY using essential oils with your partner

OILS TO AVOID

This list is based on knowledge of the general properties of the essential oils. For example, an oil that is known to thin the blood or stimulate the onset of a period should not be used in pregnancy because of the risks it could pose. The following oils should not be used during pregnancy:

• Basil
• Hyssop
• Parsley
• Pennyroyal
• Sage

ylang-ylang, grapefruit, orange, bergamot, lemon, petitgrain, frankincense, chamomile, lavender, cypress, ginger, coriander, sandalwood, pine, rose otto, and patchouli.

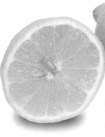

ESSENTIAL OIL of lemon is one of the safest oils to use in pregnancy

Aromatherapy aid for common conditions

• Back pain – chamomile or lavender massage
• Cramps – lavender or lemon massage
• Early morning sickness – ginger, chamomile or lavender as a room spray or in a diffuser
• Haemorrhoids – cypress and Roman chamomile in a compress
• Headaches – a few drops of diluted lavender on the forehead, or a lavender compress (see pages 24–5)
• Heartburn – ginger, lemongrass, lavender, mandarin or coriander as inhalations or in a bath
• Insomnia – chamomile or lavender in a room spray, or a few drops of neroli or lavender on a tissue on your pillow
• Low mood – lavender, neroli or geranium massage, or room spray
• Stretch marks – prevent these by massaging your tummy with essential oils of frankincense, lavender or neroli diluted in a base combination of almond and wheatgerm oils
• Tiredness – frankincense, ginger, lavender or patchouli massage, room sprays or inhalations

Six of the best

GERANIUM – good for backache, painful swollen breasts, cystitis, swollen ankles, colds, sore throats, infections. Geranium is uplifting, balancing and pain-relieving. It also improves circulation and has anti-inflammatory action.

NEROLI – good for digestive problems (constipation, diarrhoea, wind), and also for emotional problems such as stress, anxiety, depression and fear. Neroli is a natural antidepressant, sedative and digestive, but it also helps prevent stretch marks. It's an expensive oil that really comes into its own in pregnancy.

BERGAMOT – for sadness and depression, cystitis, aches and pains, and indigestion. Bergamot is pain-relieving, antibacterial and uplifting. Make sure that you buy bergamot with the bergaptene removed as otherwise it can cause sun sensitivity.

FRANKINCENSE – for stress, aches and pains, skin tone and stretch marks. Frankincense encourages deep breathing and is a great aid to meditation. It's also rejuvenating, antibacterial and comforting.

CHAMOMILE – for backache, aches and pains, headaches, wind, constipation, breast pain, cystitis and nasal congestion. Chamomile is a natural anti-inflammatory and pain reliever with calming properties to soothe a range of troubled emotions.

LAVENDER – for backache, headaches and migraines, muscle and joint pain, insomnia, coughs and colds, depression, stretch marks and infections. Another great all-rounder, lavender encourages cell renewal and relaxes muscles. It's a natural antiseptic as well as being an effective antidepressant.

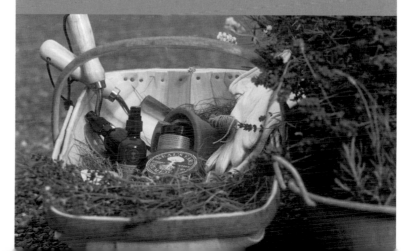

Yoga and Meditation

Inner Calm

Yoga and meditation are great ways of looking after yourself in pregnancy and preparing for the birth. Even if you've never done it before, it is safe to start now – as long as you tell your teacher you are pregnant. If you can take a dedicated pregnancy yoga class, that is even better and listen to your body so you don't do anything too strenuous.

 A lot of the yoga exercises you do in pregnancy will focus on strengthening the pelvic floor muscles (see pages 30–1). These crucial muscles support the weight of the uterus and baby, and toning them will keep them flexible and elastic so they will spring back quickly after birth. The stronger your pelvic floor muscles are, the less likely you are to experience problems such as incontinence when you sneeze or laugh, and you will also be better able to avoid an uncomfortable dragging feeling when you run, walk or even stand.

Pelvic floor muscles also play a role in delivery so being actively aware of them can help lessen the risk of a tear during delivery – but even if you do tear or need stitches, the healthier your pelvic floor is, the faster it will heal afterwards.

But there's a lot more to yoga than the pelvic floor, and the following postures, or asanas, are particularly useful in pregnancy.

Corpse

This is a lovely, deeply relaxing posture (though thankfully not quite as relaxing as the name suggests!), which involves nothing more strenuous than lying on your back on the floor. Keep your body in a nice straight line, arms by your sides (palms facing up), legs rolling out loosely from the hips, and your feet falling gently out to the side. After week 30, you may find this is less comfortable.

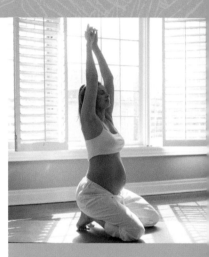

CORPSE POSTURE is deeply relaxing

LOVE YOGA

Make yoga your friend for life, not just for pregnancy. In a recent nine-week yoga study even the most basic poses and breathing exercises improved the stability and balance of older women, reducing their risk of falls. Women of all levels of health and fitness experienced remarkable benefits.

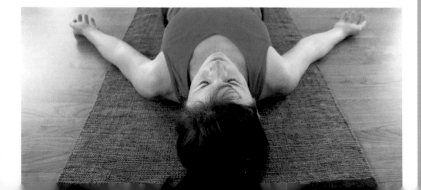

Meditation

Meditation is a great way to calm the mind. The idea is to empty it of all the cluttered thoughts that are normally in there. To do this, it's best to find a focus – try an image of a relaxing place where you feel happiest. Breathing also helps to focus the mind, and there are numerous breathing exercises you can do to ease yourself into a deep meditative state. You can meditate while lying down, or by sitting comfortably cross-legged, with your hands, palms facing down, on your knees, or knuckles down with your thumbs and first fingers touching (see opposite). Start by breathing in and out through the nose to the count of four, then, if this is comfortable, to the count of six, and finally eight, then back down to six, and four. As you breathe in, feel your diaphragm move downwards. As you breathe out, it will relax upwards. This exercise will also make more room in the abdomen and will make later pregnancy more comfortable.

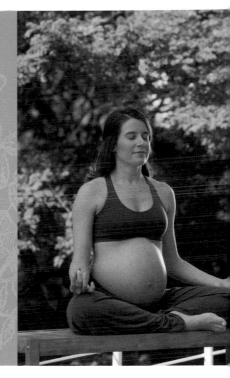

The Cat

Great for lower back pain, the 'cat' helps to loosen your spine. Start on all fours, with your knees directly in line with your hips and your wrists in line with your shoulders. As you breathe in, dip your spine, lifting your head, chest and tail. As you breathe out, reverse the posture, arching your spine as you lower your head and tuck your tail bone under. Repeat several times.

THE CAT helps maximise spine flexibility

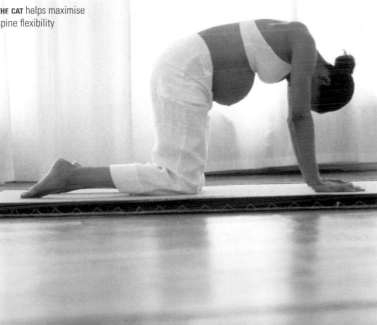

Legs up the wall

Also deeply relaxing, but again unsuitable after 30 weeks, start by sitting side on to a wall, lie down and swivel round until your legs are up the wall, with no space between your buttocks and the wall, and your back is in a neat right angle to your legs. Have a cushion under your head, if it's more comfortable, and place your hands under the tip of the back of your head (not under your neck). The position opens your chest (enabling easier breathing), relaxes tired legs and stretches out your back. If you like, you can let your legs fall gently to the side. To get out of the posture, swivel yourself side on to the wall again as you bring your legs back down.

Only hold postures for as long as is comfortable – this may be just a minute or so to start with.

Getting to Know Your Baby

Earliest Communication

From the time you first felt your baby move, you will have had an urge to keep touching your tummy – a sign of your instinctive need to bond with him or her. And just as much as you love touching your baby, your baby loves feeling you do so. He or she is quickly getting to recognise your hand, as well as your partner's – and to respond to you. You may notice the baby stops moving when an unfamiliar hand pats your tummy. Research shows that you really can get to know your baby before he or she is born, and some women are extremely tuned in to their children pre-birth.

 If you feel you'd like to get to know your baby better, start by watching for the patterns of movement and kicks from the womb. Take these as an invitation to touch him or her back. If you can't identify which part of the body is which, ask your midwife to give you a guided tour at your next appointment.

Earliest communication involves pressing gently on a spot where you have just felt a kick to see if your baby responds with another one. Later you can try giving a little massage by stroking the area covering the head, back or bottom. You can also talk to your baby – if the baby is awake, he or she will be all ears. Studies show that babies can hear fully from 20 weeks after conception; researchers, using ultrasound, have been able to see how babies react in the womb to the sounds of their parents' voices, and other sounds around them – and some babies seem to recognise their parents immediately after birth, calming down as soon as they hear their familiar voices. Babies are also fond of music with strong, regular beats, so play your favourite tunes every day. Research suggests that babies will recognise this music after they are born, and may even be calmed by it. Other studies have shown that, even in the womb, babies breathe in time to the music they enjoy. But they need variety – getting too repetitive with any activity, be it talking, singing or playing the same old tune, will just

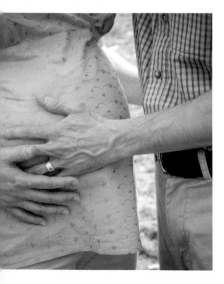

YOUR BABY will soon get to know familiar hands, even from inside the womb

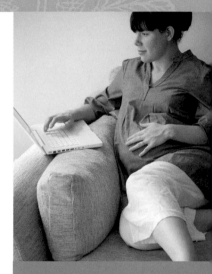

KEEP IN TOUCH

- Listen to music – see how your baby reacts.
- Watch your tummy for playful movements when you're in the bath.
- Talk softly to your baby when you know he or she is awake.
- Introduce your partner so baby gets to know his touch, too.

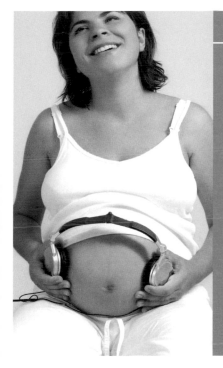

DIY DJ

A small study at Leicester University found that one-year-old babies can still recognise music they were exposed to up to three months before birth. Babies are famously exposed to Mozart or Bach in the womb – thought to stimulate the growing brain – but experts say the so-called Mozart effect is exaggerated. In the Leicester study, mothers-to-be chose a variety of different genres – including jazz, pop and reggae as well as classical. They played the music to their babies every day for the last three months before birth. More than a year later, 11 of the babies were tested and showed a preference for these pieces of music (by looking towards the source of the music) compared with very similar pieces they had not heard before. A control group of babies tested with the same music showed no preference for a particular piece. One mother who had played Ella Fitzgerald to her baby in the womb used the same Ella track to calm her baby when she awoke at 3 am – and the baby quickly settled.

cause them to tune out. Five to 10 minutes a day of dedicated baby stimulation is enough, according to studies at the Prenatal University in Hayward, California – if only to help you engage and become more attentive as parents.

Stay calm!

Everyone keeps telling you to calm down, and research shows that when a pregnant mother is tense, her baby's heart rate also increases and her movement patterns change. Other studies have shown that if you're over-anxious there's a greater likelihood of your baby being smaller than average and prone to hyperactivity. If you can make time to wind down and relax, you will be helping your baby's development – and, with luck, you will also produce a calmer child. If you find it hard to relax, book yourself a session with an aromatherapist, who can use calming oils to help you; or a reflexologist or shiatsu practitioner, who can help release tension by unblocking meridians to allow a better flow of qi energy.

TAKE TIME to enjoy inner calm – an aromatherapist can also help with this

47

The Third Trimester

The Last Three Months

You're on the final leg of your journey, but the last three months can seem the longest and most tiring. By the start of the third trimester, your baby is fully formed but growing bigger and stronger, ready for birth. His or her movements are becoming more organised and consistent, with clearly defined periods of rest and activity. For you, this is likely to be an exciting and emotional time, as well as a very body-conscious one.

 As you go through this last trimester, you may be jumpy about any niggle that could indicate an early labour – and your anxiety is likely to be exacerbated by the intensifying of your practice, or 'Braxton Hicks', contractions. Always talk your worries over with your doctor or midwife. Lower abdominal pain may be a symptom of your ligaments stretching, but if it's continuous or very bad, your midwife will be able to advise you on the best ways to support your bump.

Rest and relax as much as you can, and save your strength for your delivery. If you feel no better after resting, report this to your doctor at your next check-up. Anaemia sometimes strikes in the third trimester and some clinics check for it in the seventh month.

Encourage good sleep by making sure you don't get too overheated – your body is naturally hotter in pregnancy – so switch to a lighter-weight duvet if you're getting uncomfortable and wear breathable layers by day.

If you become shorter of breath during this trimester, because of the pressure of the uterus restricting

SLOWING DOWN is good for both of you so take every chance you have to rest in the last trimester

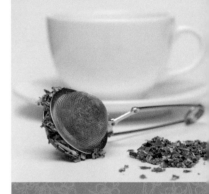

RASPBERRY LEAF TEA

Drinking raspberry leaf tea is a lovely way to strengthen and tone the uterus, making it more flexible for labour. But only drink it (up to three times a day) in the last trimester, as it has been known to over-stimulate the uterus. If your practice contractions are increasing, cut back on your dosage.

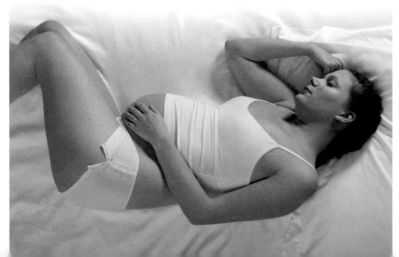

Your changing body

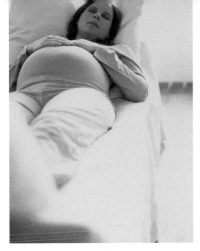

MAKE YOURSELF comfortable – extra pillows may help

your lungs and diaphragm, try adjusting your position to see if this helps. For example, if your breathing is more uncomfortable when you lie down, try propping yourself up with several pillows. However, don't ignore any severe breathlessness with rapid breathing and chest pain – this needs urgent medical attention.

Couple time

Intercourse may be difficult in the last weeks if you feel bulky and tired and can't find a comfortable position. A gentle and understanding partner can make it much easier for you – and woman on top or spooning positions tend to work best – but if you really don't feel up to sex, it's better to be honest. Maybe you can compromise with a massage that you'll both enjoy. Close to term, intercourse can help speed things along – but should not be attempted after your waters have broken, as this could introduce an infection to the uterus.

LAVENDER OIL prevents scarring and stretch marks

STRETCH MARKS

Whether you get stretch marks in pregnancy depends on whether you have an inherited tendency towards them. The stretch occurs in the collagen level of the skin and is thought to be linked to production of corticosteroids in pregnancy. The marks may appear on your abdomen, thighs, breasts and buttocks, and, although quite alarmingly reddish purple to begin with, they usually fade within six months of delivery. Regular exercise (especially walking and swimming) will improve the circulation and help keep them under control, and a daily massage with wheatgerm oil scented with a drop of neroli oil (see pages 42–3) or lavender oil will keep your skin supple and may reduce the marks.

SWELLING

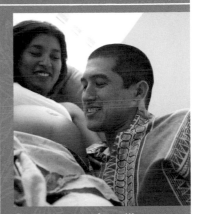

Some degree of swelling (oedema) in the feet, ankles and lower legs is considered normal in pregnancy – 75 per cent of us experience it, especially towards the end of the day, in hot weather, or if we've been standing for a long time. Usually it disappears overnight. Drinking plenty of water helps prevent water retention, but spread it through the day. If the swelling is causing you discomfort, put your legs up, wear comfortable shoes, and avoid elastic-top socks or stockings. Support tights also help, but put them on first thing in the morning, before the swelling has started. If your hands or face become puffy, tell your doctor – this could be a sign of pre-eclampsia, which needs speedy treatment.

Getting Ready for Birth

Final Preparations

As your estimated date of delivery (EDD) draws nearer, it is natural to want to do all you can to take control over the birth, and it is hugely empowering to plan ahead. There's much evidence that positive thinking can bring about what we want in life, but even if things don't go quite as perfectly as you would have liked, you will at least have spent some time focusing on the birth and engaging with your new role as a mother.

One way to take hold of the reins at this time in your pregnancy is to write a birth plan. Just setting time aside to put pen to paper is a chance to focus on the life-changing event ahead of you. You can think about who you want with you for the birth, what you want to be doing (lying, bathing or moving around), whether you want music in the background, or aromatherapy oils in the air. In case you don't feel strong enough to assert yourself in labour, you will have the whole lot written down, so that your midwife and birthing partner can carry out your wishes.

However, as many women discover, having a birth plan that, in the end, does not go according to plan can cause great disappointment – so probably the first point you should make on your plan is 'be flexible'! Yes, you hope for a natural delivery with no pain relief; yes, you would like to be at home, and with the midwife you have come to know throughout your pregnancy – but ideally, yes, you will also be able to accept a change to your plans. Midwives have lives and crises of their own, and unanticipated hitches in labour can mean you're safer in hospital. Prepare for the unexpected – and have a pain-relief contingency plan too. When it comes to it, you may not be as stoical as you imagined!

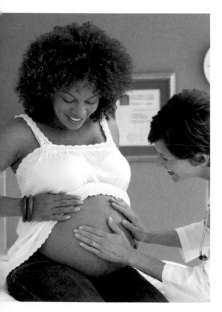

IT MAY BE hard to believe you will soon cross the border to motherhood

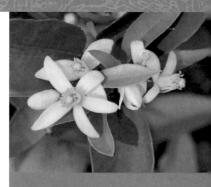

NATURAL REMEDIES

The essential oils of mandarin and orange blossom are calming at this point in your pregnancy; and the homœopathic remedy Caulophyllum (blue cohosh) can be taken from 37 weeks to strengthen contractions and soften the cervix for an easier delivery. Take one dose of Caulophyllum 30c three times a week.

PREPARE YOUR PERINEUM

Massage can help to prepare the perineum, making the area more supple, and therefore less likely to tear during birth. Use wheatgerm or almond oil daily after a warm bath, in the last eight weeks of pregnancy.

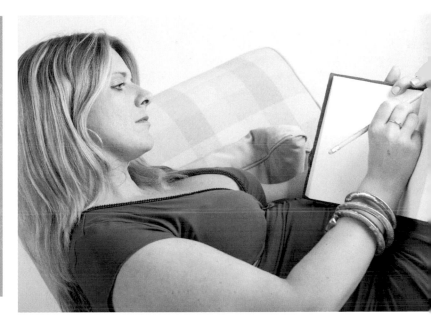

KEEP PLANS in one notebook for easy reference

YOGA FOR AN EASIER BIRTH

SQUATTING
This will help if you want to squat in labour. Squat down, keeping your back lengthened. If you can, keep your heels on the floor and balance your weight evenly between the balls of your feet and the heels, not allowing your feet to roll inward or outward. Always get up slowly, preferably holding on to a chair or table, or you may feel dizzy.

THE LAZY DOG
This is a good exercise to use to get comfortable in labour. Kneel on all fours, with a cushion under your knees if necessary. Move your pelvis from side to side like a lazy dog wagging a very heavy tail. Look round at each hip as you bring it forward, and keep your back horizontal, not curved or caving in.

WHOLE BODY RELAXATION
Relaxation, practised regularly, will prepare you for a more relaxed labour. Lie on your back on the floor and, starting with your pelvis, take one body part at a time, tense it, pressing into the floor, and then relax it. When your whole body is relaxed, your mind should slow down too.

Your birth plan
When making a birth plan, think about the following:
• Who would you like to be with you for the birth?
• Do you want to be attended by women only?
• If yours is a teaching hospital, will you mind if medical students are present?
• Do you want the freedom to move around in labour?
• Is there a special position you'd like to use for delivery?
• Do you plan to manage without pain relief?
• Do you want music in the background?
• Are you planning to use any alternative therapies for labour?

Planning a Natural Birth

Know Your Options

Childbirth is, of course, a natural process – but medical intervention can make it seem a very unnatural one. The best way to ensure that you have a delivery that is as intervention-free as possible is to plan ahead. From your earliest antenatal appointment, you should establish the facts about maternity services in your area. Ask early on about home birth services, or alternatives such as dedicated maternity units. Another option is to pay for the services of an independent midwife, who will see you throughout the pregnancy and delivery.

Many women have very strong views about what they want from their childbirth experience – and understandably so. This is possibly the most momentous event in your life. When you tell your birth story – as you will do over and over again – you'll want to remember it having gone according to your wishes. That may mean giving birth in your own home, with a midwife who has become your friend over the past few months, and the comfort of family around you. Feeling minimal pain, without drug relief,

• Who will look after your other children?
• How far do you live from the hospital?
• Is your pregnancy suitable for a home birth?
• Do you have room for a birthing pool?

is another high priority for most women, as drugs inevitably dull the experience of childbirth and will linger in your baby's system too.

If you have been looking after yourself in pregnancy – eating well, doing yoga to keep flexible, and practising relaxation to keep calm – then there's every reason to believe that your labour and delivery will go well, providing your baby is in the right position for birth (see pages 56–7) and you have no other identifiable complications. And if you are happy in your own skin, and feel you have a good connection with your baby, ultimately it may not matter where you give birth, or whether the midwife assisting you is someone you have never met before: it will be a happily memorable experience.

When things go wrong

But, as we stressed when discussing birth plans (pages 50–1), it is important to be open-minded about the birth. All the planning in the world cannot

MAKE SURE all your plans are in place

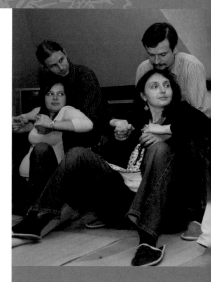

CHILDBIRTH CLASSES

Attending a dedicated childbirth class can help your chances of giving birth without intervention. Find classes from the National Childbirth Trust (www.nct.org.uk) or the Active Birth Centre (www.activebirthcentre.com).

HOME BIRTH

If you're planning on giving birth at home there's much to arrange and some research to do too. Where will you give birth? Will you be able to reach the bathroom easily? Is the room big enough for your partner and attendees? You may find that your pregnancy is considered too 'high risk' for a home birth. If this happens to you, you can ask your doctor and midwife to explain in writing why they feel this to be the case.

USING A BIRTHING POOL

Giving birth in water is relaxing and reduces pain. Check where you can hire or buy a birthing pool and which sort of pool is best suited to you and your home. The main issues are the size of the pool and the ease of connection to your hot water system. Many hospitals also offer birthing pools, but if you are afraid that it will not be available, bringing your own pool in may be an option. If a water birth is a high priority for you, do make your midwife aware of this during your antenatal clinic sessions so there is time to plan ahead.

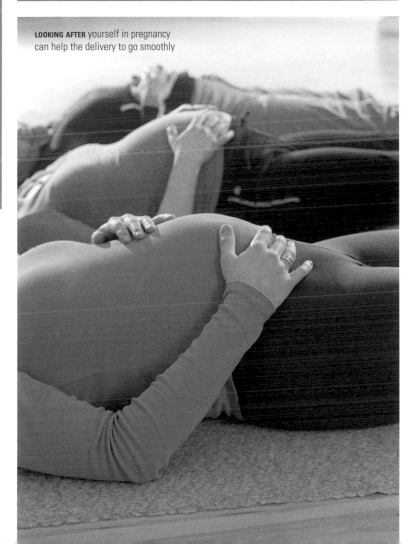

LOOKING AFTER yourself in pregnancy can help the delivery to go smoothly

prevent some babies from having to be born by caesarean section, or with forceps (or ventouse) – and many women who vowed they would not use pain relief end up having no choice because of a long and extremely difficult labour. Clearly this is not the natural birth you may have planned, but there are still steps you can take. For example, your partner can be present to massage you and help with breathing exercises. Importantly, by being flexible about what may happen, you reduce the risk both of disappointment and of depression following the birth.

The Final Countdown

Waiting For Baby

As your pregnancy moves towards its 40th week, one question will be uppermost in your mind – exactly when will your baby arrive? The window of opportunity for delivery of the nine out of ten babies that are 'on-time' is broad – four whole weeks, between the 38th and 42nd week of pregnancy. Unless you have a planned caesarean, you can only guess when your baby will enter the world. Even the best midwives and obstetricians are not fortune-tellers. However, there are a few factors that may determine whether your baby will be one side or the other of the 40th week.

 The main thing that influences a baby's arrival date is your normal menstrual cycle. When your pregnancy was confirmed, you were given an EDD calculated as 280 days from the first day of your last menstrual period. This assumes that the baby was conceived when you ovulated in that month –14 days after the start of your period, and 14 days before your next period if you have a regular (28-day) cycle. If your cycle is shorter or

MOON CYCLES may have an influence on when your baby is born

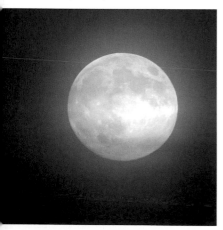

longer than 28 days, this enhances the chances of your baby coming before or after the EDD. If you want to work out exactly when your baby was conceived, there are online calculators that can help you – and some experts suggest that working out the date of your baby's conception will also give you some idea of the baby's gender, if you haven't already found out from an ultrasound scan.

Another influence is the moon. An American study that looked at half a million births over eight years in the 1960s found that more babies are born in the three days around the Full Moon than at any other time in the month. The same study found that birth takes place at the same lunar phase of the month as when conception took place – usually corresponding to the very day. It's thought sexual activity peaks around the Full Moon, while it is lowest around a New Moon – and, correspondingly, this study

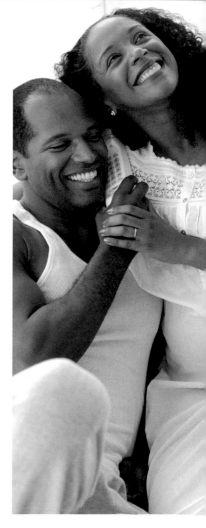

ENJOY TIME with your partner in the final weeks of pregnancy as two will soon become three

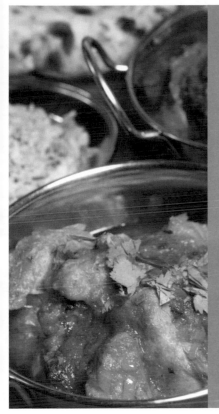

How can you kick-start labour?

The following are all known to help:

EATING CURRY
Spicy foods are great if your baby's overdue as they have a similar (though not so fierce) effect to old-fashioned castor-oil, stimulating the bowels, which in turn can help trigger the start of labour (though nobody knows exactly why).

MAKING LOVE
Semen contains natural prostaglandin. In hospital doctors often give a synthetic form of prostaglandin as a pessary if it is necessary to induce labour.

DIMMING THE LIGHTS
Your body needs to feel safe, secure and relaxed before the birth hormones can really get going so labour can progress unhindered.

HAVING YOUR NIPPLES STIMULATED!
Here's something for your partner to do. Stroking or massaging the nipples helps trigger the release of the hormone oxytocin, which helps move labour along. In trials, nipple stimulation has been proved more effective than syntocinon, the synthetic hormone administered by injection to induce contractions.

found that the smallest number of births took place in the three days around the New Moon.

So, if you are eager to predict when your baby will be born, use an online calculator to help you work out the date of conception according to the length of your menstrual cycle. Your baby is due 265 days later – but a Full Moon just before or after this date may bring your baby into the world a few days earlier or later than you expect!

Late arrival?

It's distressing to think your baby is late. The phone never stops ringing with anxious friends and relatives wanting to know how you are, and this can add to your own stress. However, studies show that 70 per

cent of babies perceived as being late are not really late at all – it is just the date of their conception that has been miscalculated. Past term, your risk of being referred for induction goes up – but this has more to do with placental deterioration than with the length of the pregnancy per se. For this reason, mothers over the age of 35 (in whom placental insufficiency is more common after 40 weeks) are more likely to have induction recommended by their doctor or midwife than are younger women.

If you are getting anxious about waiting for your baby to arrive, remember every pregnancy ends eventually – and so will yours!

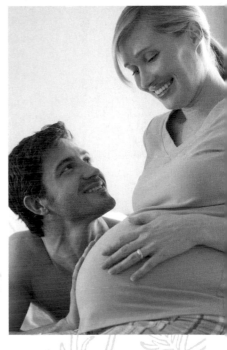

GET INTIMATE to speed your baby along

Breech Baby?

Positioned For Birth

About three per cent of babies are breech presentation – lying bottom down rather than head down at term. Although this tends to lead to a more difficult labour, many mothers do manage to successfully deliver their breech babies vaginally. Ideally, however, you will have persuaded your baby to turn around so he or she is in the cephalic (head down) position for birth. Prior to 34 weeks, the baby has ample room to turn around – and most do. But, later than this, there are natural aids that can still prompt your baby to change position.

 The majority of babies settle into a head down (cephalic) position for birth, with their chin to their chest, and spine towards their mother's back. This is the ideal position for birth, making it easiest for the baby to pass through the birth canal. If your baby is not lying correctly, it is worth trying to help him or her move into a better position. You can do this by trying to keep as active as possible throughout the pregnancy, and by walking tall – so you don't let your lower back slump into a hollow position. Slouching encourages a baby to turn into the back-to-back position, so, where possible, sit with your bottom well back in your chair, and keep your lower back supported. Sitting on a foam wedge helps even more, by tilting your pelvis forward and keeping your spine erect. If your baby is in a back-to-back or breech position, try getting on all fours for a short time every day to encourage him or her to turn. Alternatively, lie on the floor with a couple of cushions under your bottom, your knees bent and your feet flat. Stay like this for at least 10 minutes. This position creates more room in the uterus and your baby may be tempted to turn around. It is also worth seeing a homœopath, acupuncturist or osteopath – all of whom can help to turn a baby. Osteopathic treatment is also very effective at releasing tension in the muscles, ligaments and bones of the pelvis that may hinder labour and delivery.

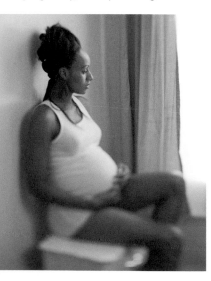

YOUR SITTING POSTURE can affect your baby's position in the uterus

ACUPUNCTURE

The Freedom Fields Hospital in Plymouth had a 60–65 per cent success rate using acupuncture to turn babies around, and some practitioners use moxibustion (using a lit 'moxa stick') to the acupoint Bladder 67 at the corner of the little toenail to help to turn the baby. It's thought to increase the number of foetal movements so that the baby somersaults into the cephalic position. If you haven't already found a good acupuncturist, see if your midwife can recommend one for you.

Baby positions

CEPHALIC – the most common presentation position – means that your baby is head down, with the top of the head (the vertex) pointing towards your cervix, and the chin tucked into the chest. This is the best position for delivery, as the narrowest part of the head is coming out first and the baby's head is protected.

BREECH – means that the baby is lying bottom-down rather than head down at term. This used to mean an automatic caesarean section, but many mothers do now successfully deliver vaginally.

BROW/FACE – means that although the baby is head down, the neck is extended so that the brow or face is pointing to the cervix. Delivered in this position, the baby may suffer some facial bruising, but this will quickly disappear. If the face is towards the cervix, delivery can be awkward and stressful for the baby. The neck can be flexed back in the process, and you may want to take the baby to a cranial osteopath in the early weeks of life.

OCCIPITO-POSTERIOR – means the back of your baby's head is facing the back of your pelvis as it comes down the birth canal. This can make labour slower and more painful – so called 'back labour'.

TRANSVERSE LIE – means the baby is lying across the womb rather than head down. If this remains the case at the start of labour, a caesarean section is unavoidable.

UNSTABLE LIE – means the baby keeps changing position between antenatal visits after 36 weeks. This could also result in a caesarean section if your baby doesn't stabilise in early labour.

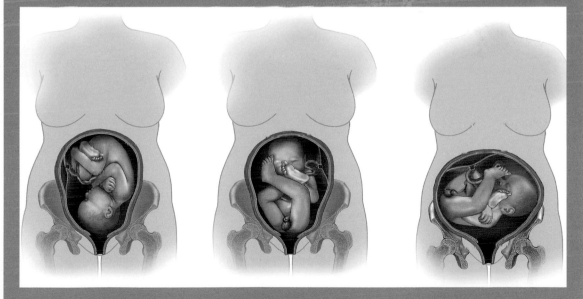

CEPHALIC BREECH TRANSVERSE LIE

Going into Labour

Is It The Real Thing?

As your due day approaches, the practice – 'Braxton Hicks' – contractions you have been having for weeks become stronger and more frequent, giving way to 'pre-labour'. This can start a full month before the real thing (or sometimes only an hour before), and is signalled by crampiness in the pelvis and rectum, persistent low backache and a change in energy levels (for better or worse). But if your contractions are intensifying and becoming more frequent, it's likely to be the real thing.

 If you think you could be in labour, call your midwife. She'll tell you what to do next. Don't be put off by fear of embarrassment in case it's not labour after all – and don't delay too long unless it's a planned home birth! Even though the start of labour may herald a long wait, it's an unpredictable process and you must be prepared for having a short labour too.

Whether you're at home or in hospital for the earliest stage of your labour, try to stay relaxed – it will help with the delivery. This is a good time to call on the relaxation exercises you've been practising. It's also a good idea to eat high-energy foods such as pasta, bananas, toast and honey, but check with your midwife as labour progresses that she's happy for you to continue eating and drinking. A warm bath is also comforting in early labour. Add essential oils of clary sage and frankincense to the water, mixed into an unscented bubble-bath base. Clary sage will tone your uterus and strengthen contractions, as well as making you feel quite euphoric. Frankincense is good for deepening your breathing, which will help you relax into the labour. Walking around can help with the pain of contractions, and squatting on a small stool between them will help open the pelvis.

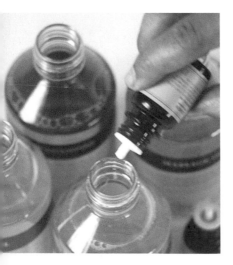

ESSENTIAL OILS added to a bubble bath base can help

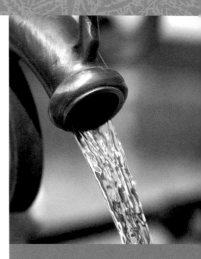

BIRTHING POOL BENEFITS

Research at the University of Liverpool found that using a birthing pool in labour led to significantly lower use of analgesic drugs, and a lower risk of both perineal tears and caesarean. It also substantially shortened the length of second stage labour (pushing).

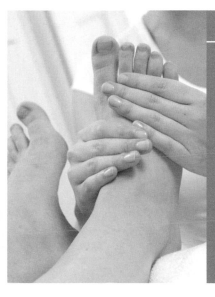

REFLEXOLOGY

A study at the Gentofte Hospital in Copenhagen found that reflexology offered outstanding pain relief for 58 out of 60 women giving birth. A further study at the Jeyrani Birth Centre, in the London borough of Newham, found that a course of 10 reflexology treatments during pregnancy could substantially reduce the length of the first stage of labour. The average in this study was five hours, compared to the textbook average of 16–24 hours. The second stage of labour took an average of 16 minutes compared to an expected 1–2 hours, and only 5.4 per cent of the women who had reflexology needed an emergency caesarean, compared to an average of 13 per cent in the area where the study was conducted.

RELAXING BREATH

Inhale slowly through one nostril, closing the other by pressing a finger against it. As you breathe in, feel your diaphragm gently rise to your chest. Breathe out, very slowly, through the opposite nostril while keeping the first one closed. As you exhale, imagine you're sending your breath through every part of your body. Continue until you feel calmer and more relaxed.

WHO'S LOOKING AFTER YOU?

Another way to maximise your chances of a quick and comfortable labour is to employ a doula – whose job is to 'mother the mother'. Doulas are experienced birth attendants with an understanding of physiology, but they are not in attendance in a clinical capacity. Their job is to offer you emotional support. In labour, your doula may help you with your breathing, relaxation and movements and she could also give you a massage. Research shows that women supported by doulas have shorter labours and lower rates of epidural and caesarean deliveries. Their babies are also less likely to suffer foetal distress or need neonatal intensive care.

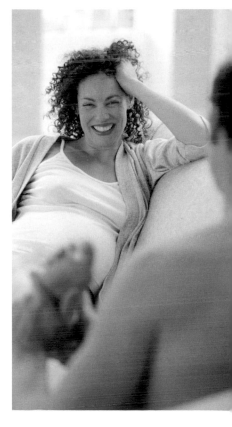

WOMEN who receive massage and comfort during labour tend to have shorter labours

Complementary therapies for pain relief

ACUPUNCTURE

HOW IT WORKS
Western doctors believe acupuncture works by triggering the release of endorphins, the body's natural painkillers; however, the Chinese view is that it simulates the flow of qi energy, thus releasing blockages causing pain.

PROFESSIONAL HELP OR DIY?
Professional: Some midwives are trained in acupuncture, and some acupuncturists will attend a birth.

ACUPRESSURE

HOW IT WORKS
This is a needle-free version of acupuncture.

PROFESSIONAL HELP OR DIY?
DIY: Your birthing partner can use the balls of his or her thumbs to apply weight to the acupoint Bladder 23 (ask an acupuncturist to show you the correct location before you go into labour). For painful back labour, apply strong finger pressure to just below the centre of the ball of the foot.

AROMATHERAPY

HOW IT WORKS
The combination of essential oils and massage is an excellent way to relieve back pain and relax you generally.

PROFESSIONAL HELP OR DIY?
DIY: Make yourself a special labour oil by combining 8 drops of jasmine absolute and 4 drops of clary sage essential oil into 30 ml of massage base oil. Ask your partner to massage it into your lower back during labour.

FLOWER REMEDIES

HOW IT WORKS
Flower remedies will relax you and lift your mood. Combine them with other forms of pain relief.

PROFESSIONAL HELP OR DIY?
Both: Seek advice from a therapist on the remedies to use, and take them with you to your birthing room, or sip a glass of water with a few drops of Bach Five Flower remedy added to it – this can be very calming in labour.

HERBALISM

HOW IT WORKS
Herbs act as powerful medicines and are a good alternative to analgesics.

PROFESSIONAL HELP OR DIY?
Both: Consult a herbalist for tailored advice, or use the following herbs during labour. Every 30 minutes, take one cupful of raspberry leaf tea with 20 drops of squaw vine tincture added. To encourage the cervix to dilate, take 10 drops of blue cohosh tincture in a little water every 30 minutes. If the contractions are weak or ineffective, then take 10 drops of golden seal tincture in a little water every 20 minutes (golden seal should not be taken during pregnancy until labour commences).

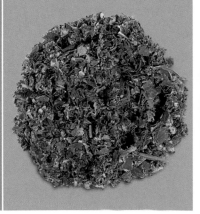

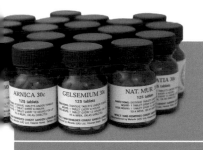

HOMŒOPATHY

HOW IT WORKS
Many remedies have specific uses that make them invaluable during labour.

PROFESSIONAL HELP OR DIY?
Both: Seek advice from a homœopath before you go into labour, and have your remedies handy. Helios Homœopathics make an excellent childbirth kit that also contains a useful leaflet. For fearfulness and anxiety during labour, try Aconite 30c or 200c; for exhaustion during a long labour, try Carbo veg 30c. When contractions are weak, try Caulophyllum 30c or 200c. If you're anxious and your contractions are unproductive, try Gelsemium 30c or 200c; if you're irritable and weepy, and your labour pains are weak, try Pulsatilla 30c or 200c; if your labour pains are unbearably, agonizingly painful, try Chamomilla 200c.

HYPNOTHERAPY

HOW IT WORKS
Hypnotherapy has been shown in studies to be more effective in childbirth than some of the strongest painkillers, including pethidine. It involves visualisation, which enables you to mentally turn down the intensity of the pain, like turning down the heat of the cooker. Some women can even turn off the pain completely.

PROFESSIONAL HELP OR DIY?
Both: Seek professional advice first. A good hypnotherapist should be able to write you an individual programme during pregnancy, which will be automatically triggered once labour starts. However, not everyone is good at self-hypnosis and you may find it difficult to concentrate.

REFLEXOLOGY

HOW IT WORKS
It works on the same meridians and qi flow as acupuncture, and improves breathing and deepens relaxation.

PROFESSIONAL HELP OR DIY?
Both: A professional reflexologist in attendance at the birth will be able to respond to your changing needs by treating specific points on your feet or hands. For relaxation in labour, your partner can also work on your hands, applying gentle thumb pressure to the dip in your palm just below the fleshy pad beneath your middle finger. This pressure should be applied in time with your in-breaths and released with your out-breaths. Massaging the crease of the joint at the base of your thumb on each hand will help to calm your mood and ease tension around your shoulders and neck.

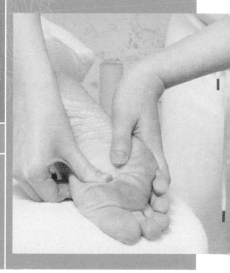

A Joint Venture

Becoming Parents Together

As a couple, your pregnancy and childbirth experiences are a chance to become even closer to each other, yet they can seem to separate many partners. Men who feel ostracised by their partner's pregnancy, or left out of things, may find it hard to express their feelings – resulting in their partner feeling rejected too. Make sure you both resolve any problems before resentment grows and risks spoiling what should be one of the best experiences of both of your lives.

 While a woman is visibly pregnant, suffering the symptoms and coping with the pain of childbirth, her partner can – in theory – carry on as if nothing is changing. Indeed, this used to be the way that most men operated. But the growing availability of paternity leave is testament to the changes that have taken place in the last 10 or 20 years. Far more men become actively involved in the pregnancy these days, and putting time into working at empathising with your pregnant partner will enable you to feel more involved from the beginning, and help to open up conversations about worries that either of you may have. As the non-pregnant partner, there is no reason that you cannot share, and enjoy, many of the following crucial experiences.

Attending obstetrician appointments

Accompany your partner to her doctor as often as you can – but especially for the landmark appointments, such as screenings and tests.

Acting pregnant

You may have trouble justifying the need for an afternoon nap, but it will be encouraging for your partner if you do her exercises with her. Giving up favourite junk food, alcohol, caffeine and cigarettes with her will also make her feel less isolated from you – and give you some idea of what she is feeling.

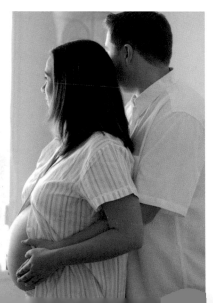

YOUR PARTNER can feel isolated if you don't make an effort to join in

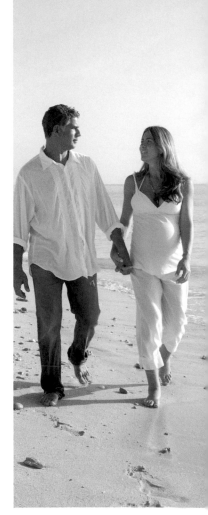

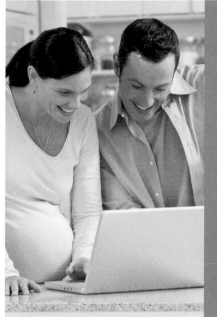

Dad's dilemma

Q. I don't want to attend the birth – will it really matter if I'm not there?

A. Your partner needs your support in childbirth, but that needn't mean being present for the delivery if you are absolutely sure that your presence will be counter-productive. If you can't be there all the way through, talk it over with your partner first. Help her find another birthing partner – a friend, relative or a doula, who can offer her the support she needs – but let her know that you are there for her emotionally, if not physically. Stay with her during the labour, so she has your hand to hold. Try to give her any comfort you can. If you still need to slip out as the baby is born, return to the room as soon as possible so you can meet your baby together – those earliest minutes as a family are precious and you will want to remember them.

Swotting up

Read as much as you can about pregnancy and childbirth, and ask friends and colleagues about their experiences too. Your partner may feel as if the burden of responsibility is on her shoulders alone, but the more informed you are, the more that burden is shared – and you will also be able to offer another perspective on any worries that she may have.

Shopping for a layette

Taking an active part in choosing nursery equipment is important – and a fun experience for you to share as a couple.

Keep on talking

Talk about the present – how you both feel today, in this moment – and the future too. You are months, weeks or days away from becoming parents. How do you see the next 12 months, five years

and even 10 years? If you feel that either one of you is avoiding talking openly for any reason, gently try to find out why that is. Is there a fear that something will go wrong with the baby? If so, it is as important to voice these painful feelings as it is to express your excitement. If you feel that you need extra help, book a session with a couples' counsellor who can help you to open up and maybe see things from another point of view.

Few of us are born to be natural mothers or fathers – instead we learn on the job. Acknowledge any anxieties you may have that you won't be a good enough parent. They are normal feelings, and it will help your partner face up to her worries about new motherhood if you can also share your concerns about your role. The more you can

talk openly with each other, the more you can both be reassured that you are doing your best as parents, and as a new family.

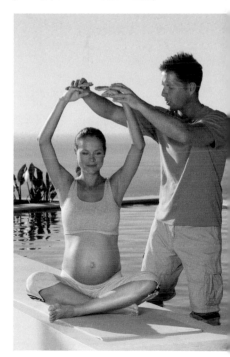

TAKING CARE of your partner can make you feel more involved in the pregnancy

If Something Goes Wrong

Addressing Our Fears

You've eaten well, taken the right kind of exercise, been good to yourself, and you deserve a happy ending – an uncomplicated delivery and a healthy baby. But, however well you look after yourself, things can still go wrong. From a much-wanted home birth being cancelled for emergency hospitalisation to the tragic loss of a baby due to stillbirth, we have to accept that some things are beyond our control. You need all the moral support you can get from your partner, and other relatives and friends. But there are also some extremely helpful remedies to help you through a difficult time.

 The worst-case scenario for any mother-to-be is the thought of her baby dying before or during labour. For a few women, this is the tragic outcome of their pregnancy: 17 babies are stillborn or die shortly after birth every day in the UK. If this should happen to you, allowing yourself to experience the grief will be the only way to emerge from such a life trauma, but there are several things that can be done to assist the grieving process. The first is to be allowed to see or hold your dead baby, thereby having a person to remember, rather than an intangible nightmarish experience. Build this requirement into your birth plan if you think there's any risk that you wouldn't be given this option. As a society we shy away from talking about death, and what happens if someone dies – however, it is much better to prepare yourself by asking your midwife how the process is handled locally. Talking about it will not bring bad luck – but it may help you cope by preparing you in a practical, if not emotional, way.

Therapies that can help

Your body will have to readjust, too, from the physical build-up of pregnancy – and taking an infusion of sage three times a day can help to stop your breasts making unneeded milk. The homœopathic remedy Lac caninum will have a similar effect. Take one dose of 200c and repeat a couple of days later if you need to.

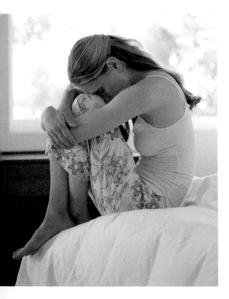

GIVE YOURSELF time and space to grieve

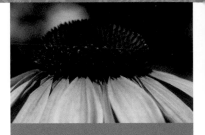

HELPFUL HEALING

HOMŒOPATHIC REMEDIES:
- Lac caninum
- Arnica
- Bellis perennis

HERBS:
- Comfrey
- Echinacea
- Marigold
- Marshmallow
- Raspberry leaf

ESSENTIAL OILS:
- Clary sage
- Lavender
- Melissa
- Neroli
- Rose

COPING WITH A CAESAREAN

Having a caesarean is the antithesis to a natural delivery for women who want less medical intervention. It also raises the risk of maternal mortality by 400 per cent and is more likely to result in infection in the mother and breathing difficulties for the baby. However, it is sometimes an unavoidable way of saving your child's life. And if you do have to have a caesarean section, there are lots of natural remedies that you can use afterwards to lessen the impact of such a major operation. Herbs to take internally to promote healing and reduce the chance of an infection include comfrey, echinacea, marigold, marshmallow and raspberry leaf. These may be combined and taken as a decoction (or as tinctures) three times a day for up to a month after the birth. Taking homœopathic Arnica straight after the operation will also help to prevent infection and promote healing. Take either a couple of doses of 200c or one 30c dose a day for five days. Bellis perennis is also very useful to relieve discomfort and speed tissue healing. Take 30c a day for five days following the Arnica. Being open-minded about birth can also make having a caesarean less of a blow.

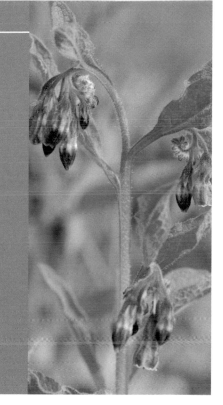

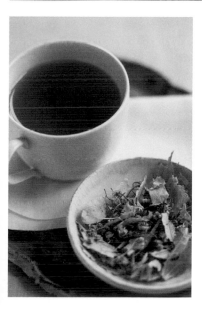

You may be offered drugs such as antidepressants or tranquillisers to help you cope with your grief, but these only tend to delay the grieving process. Bach Five Flower Remedy can be taken several times a day during an emotional crisis; and the homœopathic remedy Ignatia is also helpful. Calming herbs for this highly stressful time include balm, chamomile, oats, skullcap and vervain, which you can combine in an infusion to drink up to three times a day. The essential oils of clary sage, lavender, melissa, neroli and rose are also mildly sedative and antidepressive. Choose one or two of these and burn them in your room, add them to your bath water or use them in a massage oil.

Professional counselling is also hugely beneficial after the loss of a baby, and both you and your partner should attend – together or separately or a mixture of both – if possible.

HERBS are a great alternative to antidepressants

Post-partum

New Mum

Whether this is your first or fourth baby, the earliest minutes and hours with your child will be etched on your memory for ever. Understandably, all you may want to do is hold your baby, and stare at him or her in wonder – so ask the midwife if you can spend some time with your baby before the essential work of checking him or her over is carried out. It's an essential part of your bonding process and a chance for you to assert your wishes as a confident, natural mother.

A lovely way to bond with your baby immediately after birth is to dim the lights and look into his or her eyes, observing the reaction you get. Your partner can share this – and there is no reason why he shouldn't also cut the cord. It is a simple enough procedure, and whether this is a home or hospital birth, you can ask your midwife to guide you if you're nervous. It's often routine procedure to clamp and cut the cord as soon as the baby is born, and to give the mother an injection of ergometrine or syntometrine to contract the uterus and expel the placenta. However, this speeding up of the third stage of labour can increase the incidence of retained placenta and maternal blood loss. Clamping the umbilical cord before it stops pulsating also has the disadvantage of depriving the baby of blood that is rightly its own.

If you have agreed to have ergometrine or syntometrine, the umbilical cord will have to be clamped after the drug is administered, to prevent the baby getting too much blood too quickly and then developing jaundice. But if you have not, then the clamping and cutting of the cord can be delayed until after the placenta has been delivered – as long as you hold your baby by your thigh, level with the placenta. This is a natural way to aid the delivery, and remaining in a squatting or kneeling

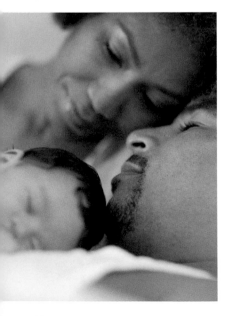

MAKE SURE YOUR partner gets a chance to have early contact with the baby as well

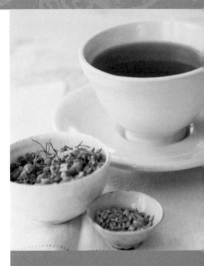

BE PREPARED

Your baby's been safely delivered, but has the placenta? If you've been using and enjoying herbal remedies during pregnancy, why not also stock up on herbs that can be used post-partum to aid the delivery of the placenta? Fresh leaf teas and herbal tinctures can be particularly helpful.

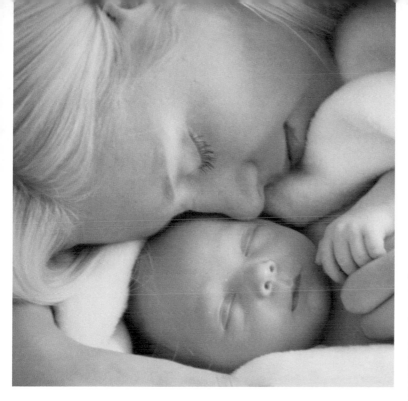

THE FIRST HOURS provide precious bonding time – make the most of them

Retained placenta

If you're unfortunate enough to have a retained placenta – which means it did not separate and deliver spontaneously – a massage with jasmine oil may help it to separate. The homœopathic remedies Caulophyllum 200c or Pulsatilla 200c can also help. Acupuncture and cranial osteopathy can help too, but you would need a practitioner on hand very quickly for these to be realistic options.

HAEMORRHAGE

Losing more than 500 ml (¾ pint) blood within 24 hours of delivery counts as post-partum haemorrhage, which is serious and potentially life threatening. Homœopathic remedies may be given while waiting for other medication to take effect or before resorting to a transfusion.

The following remedies are the most likely to help: arnica (if the haemorrhage is due to lacerations), caulophyllum (if the uterus is too weak to contract, after an arduous labour), ipecac (if the bleeding is sudden and profuse), or sabina (if the blood is dark and there are severe pains in the uterus).

position allows gravity to speed things along.

Babies are often born ready to suck – and not only is it a lovely feeling to put your baby straight to the breast, the sucking will also stimulate contractions to release the placenta. But don't try to force it if it doesn't feel right. Not all babies want to suck straight away, and, from a bonding point of view, it is just as lovely to hold your baby close to your breast – skin on skin. This will also get them used to the idea of the breast, for feeding. If your partner strokes your nipples, this will have the same effect on contractions.

If delivery of the placenta seems slow, there are some herbs that can help. Ask your partner to make you a decoction of angelica root, raspberry leaf and shepherd's purse (one cup is usually enough,

although another may be taken half an hour later if you need it); or try black or blue cohosh, also as a decoction (one cup) or 20 drops of tincture in a little water.

BLACK COHOSH is used to relax the uterine muscles and may still have a role to play post-partum

The First Six Weeks

Make Time For You

Your instinct is to nurture and pamper your baby in his or her earliest weeks of life – but this is a time when you need to be well looked after, too. You have the physical as well as the emotional readjustment to make, and by accepting and addressing your own needs as well as those of your baby, you maximise your chances of becoming a confident mother, with the energy needed to fulfil your task with ease.

This is a time when you may feel least inclined to put yourself first – your baby is uppermost in your mind. But remember the instructions you're given when you're on a plane – 'always put on your own oxygen mask before helping someone else with theirs'. As a brand new mother, you also need your own supply of oxygen – emotional and physical nurturing – in order to give yourself optimally to your baby.

We can think of no better excuse to curl up with your baby while other people do the household chores and bring you food and drink! If you have the luxury of friends and family willing to help you out, make the most of it. If you have taken on the services of a doula, this is exactly the kind of practical help she can provide. In many cultures it is *de rigueur* to tuck a new mother up with her baby for the first few weeks – so they can devote themselves to bonding. This is a simple and natural indulgence that you should not feel guilty about enjoying.

To help your recovery, try the Chinese herb dang gui (Chinese angelica). It has been used by thousands of women over the centuries in China to restore energy and tonify the blood and reproductive organs following childbirth and is worth taking as a tincture (2 ml in water three times a day).

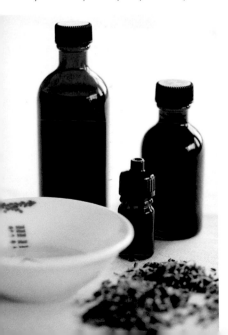

DON'T COMPROMISE – always invest in top quality herbs and tinctures

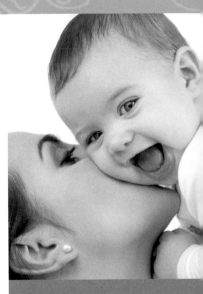

THIS IS A TIME FOR...

- Keeping your days simple and stress-free.
- Bonding with your baby.
- Letting yourself be looked after.
- Forgetting that you are normally the one who runs the household.
- Enjoying being a mum.

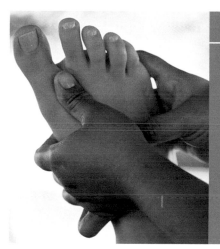

Lochia is the name given to the vaginal bleeding you experience after childbirth. For the first 48 hours it's likely to be quite heavy – much heavier than any period you have experienced – and you will need to use large maternity pads. After the first two days the blood loss lessens, but altogether it will continue for anything from two to six weeks after the birth. Talk to your midwife if you have any concerns about it but a useful tip to help control excessive lochia is by applying pressure to a reflexology point just in front of the webbing between your big toe and the one next to it on the upper side of your right foot.

The following remedies will also aid your physical recovery in the first six weeks:

Afterpains

The homœopathic tissue salt Mag phos 6X can be taken every few hours for up to five days to ease any afterpains (contractions caused by the uterus returning to its normal size). If the pains are very severe, and particularly if they make you feel irritable, try homœopathic Chamomilla 30c. A herbal combination that relieves afterpains and also helps the uterus to readjust can be made from black cohosh, blue cohosh, crampbark and raspberry leaf. (Make a decoction to drink three times a day for a few days, or use tinctures). Alternatively, add a few drops of the antispasmodic essential oils of chamomile, lavender or marjoram pre-diluted in base oil to a warm bath, or apply to your abdomen as a warm compress.

CALENDULA is wonderfully soothing next to the skin

Bruising

Calendula tincture is useful for bruising. Soak a sanitary pad in diluted tincture of calendula, which is very soothing, freeze it and then wear it next to your skin until it thaws out.

Arnica is helpful to relieve any bruising and promote healing after the trauma of birth. Take Arnica 30c three times a day for a week.

Coccyx pain

St John's wort can help with pain in your tailbone (the coccyx) if it was pushed backwards as the baby passed through the birth canal.

Although St John's wort is best known as a natural antidepressant, herbalists also recommend it for chronic nerve pains and for trauma and injury involving nerve damage. If the problem lasts longer than a few days, an osteopath should be able to relieve it.

ARNICA can be used to promote healing after birth

Taking care of your baby and yourself

Devoting time to recovering from the birth and bonding with your new baby will help you learn to listen to – and trust – your maternal instinct. For many mothers, this is something that does not come easily, despite what you may imagine when you see other women with their babies. Remember – appearances can be deceptive, and to others you too may look as if you've taken to motherhood like a duck to water when, beneath the surface, only you know how frantically your feet are paddling to stay afloat!

As well as investing in your physical recovery, it's worth taking steps to help yourself adjust emotionally too. Make time for meditation, which is a great way to calm an anxious mind and put muddled thoughts in order. Flower remedies can also be very grounding, and a visit to a flower remedy therapist could prove very worthwhile in the first six weeks. Some especially useful Bach Flower Blends include S.O.S. if you are feeling overwhelmed and panicky, Revitalise if you are feeling shattered and Optimism if you are suffering with the 'baby blues'.

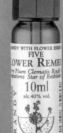

FLOWER REMEDIES can help with emotional issues

BABY BLUES

After months of looking forward to your baby's arrival, a few days after birth it can suddenly seem that everything is wrong, even though nothing actually is. What you are experiencing is the 'baby blues'. It is more than an emotional reaction to the birth – it has a physical trigger: the change in hormone levels after delivery. Throughout pregnancy, hormone levels rise to accommodate the baby and, by the time labour begins, levels of progesterone and oestrogen are 50 times higher than they were before the pregnancy. After the birth, these levels fall suddenly and dramatically to below the levels they were at before the pregnancy began. The good news is that this feeling should pass within a few hours or, at the most, a few days.

In the meantime you need to be given the freedom to cry and express your fluctuating emotions. If you feel miserable you should not be told to pull yourself together, but instead listened to and reassured that the misery will soon pass. Empathy and tact are all important at this time.

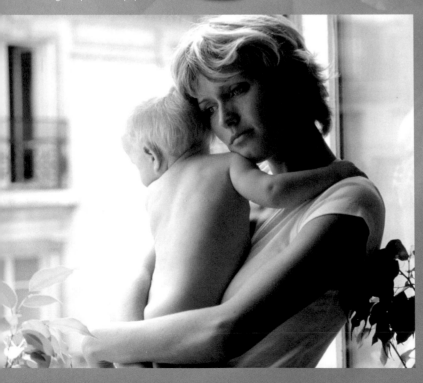

ENJOY YOUR BABY

This is a time when babies and their mothers belong together. Instead of leaving your baby alone sleeping in an upstairs room, take him round the house with you in a crib or a sling so he can be seen and heard at all times, especially when he cries. This will usually be because of hunger – and if you are nearby, your baby won't be kept waiting! You can't spoil a baby by picking him up and devoting time to him; and, by going to your baby whenever he needs attention, you will help him to feel loved and secure. Think of every cuddle being a boost to his growing confidence!

At night, your baby can sleep in your room, so he can easily be fed. Keeping night feeds low-key, for example, and changing the nappy with minimal fuss (a baby sleeping bag or nightie will allow you easy access) will minimise the disruption to your night. Once a baby is too big for a crib, and is beginning to sleep through most nights, then you can think about moving him into a cot in a separate room. At six weeks old there is no rush for a baby to grow up!

BONDING TIME FOR DADS

If you are breastfeeding – and especially if this is taking up much of your time in the early weeks – your partner may find it hard not to feel marginalized by the baby. Instead of using him solely as your servant to run around catching up with chores or looking after older children while you and the baby chill out, encourage him to have bonding time with the baby too. Hand the baby over when she is awake and can be cuddled and talked to by your partner while you take a bath or shower, or make him a cup of tea – don't save all these things for when the baby is asleep, with her 'do not disturb' sign up! It's healthy for you to relinquish control of the baby too, so quietly observe how your partner interacts with her. You may discover things you never knew about your partner, and your baby.

GETTING TO KNOW YOUR BABY

In the first two weeks babies are awake only 10 per cent of the time, and when they are, they may be looking around quietly ('quiet alert'), gradually focusing on your face. This is a great time to bond as you notice your baby take in a little bit more of your face every day. By week five, he or she will turn towards a bell you ring, or a toy that you squeak – make the most of these early play times.

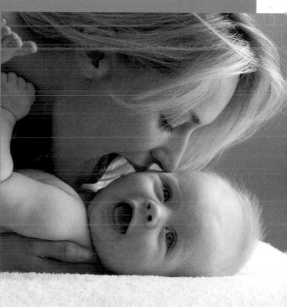

Breastfeeding

New Skills

There is nothing more natural than breastfeeding your baby, and, when you do so, you provide your baby with a warm, fresh, sterile and conveniently available feed that is easily digestible, and full of antibodies and anti-allergens to protect your baby from disease and infection. And if that's not enough, there are also benefits for you too. Some believe you will speed up the process of shedding pregnancy weight, while also enjoying gorgeous closeness with your baby.

All through pregnancy your breasts have been preparing to feed your new baby – and the first feed can take place straight after birth. The longer and more frequently your baby sucks, the sooner your milk will 'come in'. Until that time, colostrum (which is rich in protein, minerals, vitamin A and nitrogen) supplies all the water and nourishment your baby needs. Colostrum contains antibodies to protect your newborn against a wide range of infections, diseases and allergies, and is the most important feed you will give your baby.

Breasts naturally produce milk according to your baby's demands – more frequent suckling at the breast stimulates more milk to be produced. Breast milk also supplies all your baby's nutritional needs up to six months and three quarters of their needs for up to a year.

To make it an optimal feed for your baby:
• Make sure your diet contains plenty of fresh fruit and vegetables, whole grains and protein-rich foods (soya beans, cheese, lentils, lean meat, fish, eggs and nuts).
• Do not attempt to crash diet as this will diminish your milk supply.
• Sugar and refined carbohydrates (such as white flour) are best avoided now too.
• Try to drink at least 2 litres (3¹/₂ pints) of water a day.

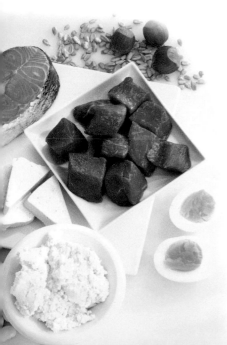

A HEALTHY DIET is good for you and your breastfed baby

Why breastfeed?

• Your breasts have an amazing ability to manufacture according to the season, so in hot weather your milk will quench his extra thirst without compromising on the food part of his feed.

• Breast milk protects your baby from allergies, infections and even obesity.

• Your baby's nappies won't be as smelly as those of a formula-fed baby.

• It's cheaper and more convenient than feeding with a bottle.

• It provides extra closeness, which adds to the bonding process between you and your baby.

If you can't breastfeed

Nearly all women can breastfeed – but breastfeeding is contraindicated if you have a serious infection or need drugs that will pass through your milk to the baby. If you cannot feed your baby, try not to feel guilty about it. Instead, make bottle feeding as enjoyable an experience as you can for both of you (and your partner, who can participate fully). Cow's milk is best avoided by babies as it is a common cause of allergies, mucus congestion and colic; so look for a goat's milk infant formula. This is much closer in nature to human breast milk and better tolerated.

CHOOSE a goat's milk formula if you can't breastfeed

Helpful remedies

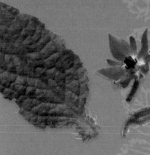

BORAGE is an herb that can help with milk supply

• For poor milk supply: make an infusion of aniseed, borage, fennel and holy thistle and drink a cupful two or three times a day for a few weeks.

• For a breastfed baby with colic, drink an infusion made from dill seeds before each feed.

• For hard and painful engorgement, take homœopathic Bryonia, or make a compress with a few drops of essential oils of chamomile, geranium, lavender or rose in warm water.

• For cracked nipples, dilute tinctures of marigold and St John's Wort in a little boiled and cooled water and dab onto the nipples after each feed.

• Mastitis is an inflammation of the breast that can develop when breastfeeding.

The symptoms are heat and redness in the breast and you may feel 'fluey' or generally unwell. Mastitis must be treated properly to prevent a serious infection developing and if it persists for more than eight hours or you get a fever then seek urgent medical advice. For mild mastitis, apply a paste of marigold and slippery elm (mix the powdered herbs with water) to the breast and leave it for a couple of hours to reduce inflammation; and take echinacea to reduce the risk of infection. Homœopathic remedies can be very effective in the treatment of mastitis. The most common remedies are: Belladonna 30c, for symptoms of heat and redness (try this first); Bryonia 30c for heaviness and fullness in the breast; and Phytolacca 30c for sharp pains and heat in the breast. In each case, take the remedy every two hours until the symptoms have gone.

• To help the weaning process, both you and your baby can take the Bach flower remedy walnut for a smoother transition.

• To help dry up milk supply, drink a sage infusion three times a day; or take a one-off dose of the homœopathic remedy Lac caninum 200c.

New Mum's Diet

Look After Yourself

Don't be swayed by the boom of celebrity mums competing to be fastest to get their pre-pregnancy figures back. In the post-natal period your body needs all the nourishment it can get – and this is no time to crash diet. Breastfeeding itself demands a lot of your energy -- you actually need 500 more calories than usual at this time – and on its own it is an effective way to get back to your pre-pregnancy weight. This is also a period when a healthy diet is vital to keep your mood stable and prevent post-natal depression.

Diet is paramount when you're looking after yourself in the first few weeks and months as a mother. Food supplements cannot take the place of a good diet with nutritious, full-of-vitality foods, but they can help to compensate and top up any shortcomings, so consider taking a good multivitamin and mineral supplement daily. Try to eat a wide range of nutritious foods every day, and including the following superfoods:

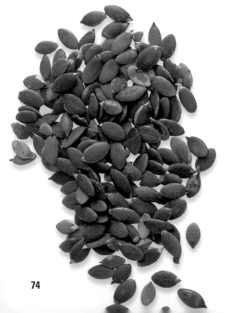

KEEP DEPRESSION at bay with essential fatty acids from seeds

Fish

Fish, which is a great source of protein and – if it's one of the oily fish (tuna, sardines, herring, mackerel and trout) – a rich source of omega 3 essential fatty acids, DHA (docosahexaenoic acid) and EPA (eicosapentaenoic acid). DHA is particularly important for the brain and nervous system, and will help to boost your mood at a time when you can easily feel low because of hormonal fluctuations, tiredness, and simply the adjustment you have to make to motherhood.

Seeds

Seeds will provide you with the essential fatty acids needed to prevent depression. Sunflower and sesame seeds are rich in calcium and magnesium, and the latter helps each cell in the body to produce energy while also working as a 'calming' mineral. Both seeds are also great sources of zinc, which boosts immunity and helps prevent depression, and the

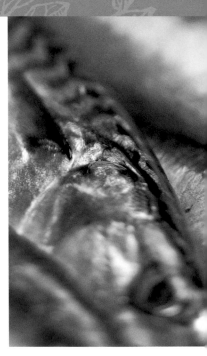

vitamin B5 they additionally contain is essential for a healthy response to stress. Sprinkle them on salads and make sure you chew the sesame seeds thoroughly to get their full benefits (because of their size, they are often left undigested). Pumpkin seeds are also worth including in your diet as they're a source of vitamin B6, which helps hormonal balance.

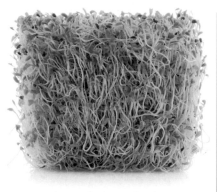

DISCOVER the superfood properties of sprouts

Sprouts

Alfalfa and mung bean sprouts, which you can grow in a propagator (from health food stores), are highly nutritious and a great addition to any salad. During sprouting, the activity of enzymes increases dramatically, effectively predigesting the seed so that it's easier for your body to break down and absorb the nutrients.

Oats

Oats are often recommended by herbalists to calm anxiety and depression, because they're loaded with B vitamins, vitamin E, and iron and zinc, all of which contribute to a healthy nervous system.

Brown rice

Brown rice, which should be cooked long enough to be chewy rather than al dente, contains vitamins, minerals, essential fatty acids and dietary fibre – much of which is lost in the process that transforms it into white rice. Its fibre slows down the release of starch as sugar into the bloodstream, making it a perfect low GI food. This balances your moods and controls cravings, and provides a satisfying and steady release of energy.

Get juicing

As a new mother, you need a strong immune system and plenty of energy, and freshly squeezed juices can help with both. Be adventurous and try the following:

BEETROOT JUICE – which has particular benefits on blood pressure. If you ended your pregnancy with hypertension, drinking a 600-ml (1-pint) glass a day will help to lower it, according to a recent study. Beetroot is also loaded with iron and beta carotene and vital for healthy blood.

CARROT JUICE – known as the 'miracle juice' – is a gold mine of nutrients. It's one of the richest sources of vitamin A (50,000 units in a 225-ml/8-oz glass) that can be used in the daily diet, as well as being a good source of B vitamins, calcium, copper, magnesium, potassium, phosphorus, chlorine, sulphur and iron.

WHEATGRASS JUICE – an amazing energiser. Wheat sprouts contain four times more folic acid and six times more vitamin C than unsprouted wheat or ordinary grass. They're too fibrous to be digested whole by humans, but, as a juice, their nutrients are completely assimilated by the body in 20 minutes. A 60-ml (2-oz) glass of fresh juice provides the equivalent in vitamins and minerals of 1.4 kilos (3 lbs) of organic vegetables, so you'll feel refreshed and energized throughout the day. Wheatgrass juice has benefits for nearly every part of the body – from blood and bones to major organs.

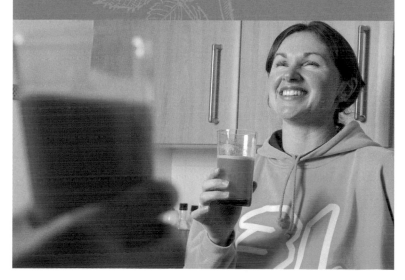

Sleep Solutions

The New Mum's Holy Grail

Some newborn babies seem to be almost permanently asleep, only waking for feeds. Others rarely seem to shut their eyes. If your baby falls into the latter category, you're also unlikely to get the sleep you need. As a new mother, you need all the energy you can get – so finding a solution to your baby's sleep problem is likely to be paramount. But babies are not failures if they are non-sleepers – and stressing about wakefulness will only further deplete your own energy stores.

 Newborn babies do not know that they are supposed to be asleep at night and awake during the day, so the first thing you can do as a mother is to show them that night time is not play time. Keep any feeds or nappy changes very low key, with minimal talk, no play, and the lights kept low. If your baby is next to your bed, it will be easy to pick him or her up for a feed without becoming fully awake yourself; and a CD of womb music or white noise may help both of you get back to sleep quickly after the feed.

What to do if your baby won't sleep

If your baby is a diehard non-sleeper, your attempts at establishing a night routine may be in vain. It's worth exploring the possibility that your baby could have an allergy that is keeping him or her awake. Torsion on the brain, caused by the pressure of birth, is another possible cause for sleeplessness. It sounds scary, but is something cranial osteopaths see all the time, and they can often solve the problem – and the baby's sleeplessness – with just one treatment.

If you have the luxury of being able to 'nest' with your baby during the early weeks, you can take any opportunity to sleep when he or she does, instead of seizing that time to rush around getting on with work. If not, do what you can to ease your own stress so that you maximise your chances of sleeping when you can, and try the following:

• Look at your diet. If you're breastfeeding, a tryptophan-rich

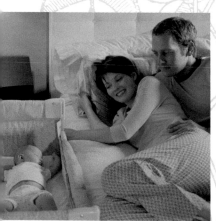

IF YOUR BABY sleeps next to your bed, it is easy to do a feed without fully waking up

SLEEPING TOGETHER

One large survey found that 50 per cent of parents sleep with their baby in their bed. Providing you are not under the influence of drugs or alcohol this should be safe, but the best safety advice is to have your baby close by your bed in his or her own crib.

diet (see pages 26–7) will help you sleep – and the foods should have a knock-on effect for your baby too. By the same token, avoid any foods that are likely to excite your baby or keep him or her awake – such as caffeine (including chocolate), spicy foods and alcohol. Also, try taking a good multivitamin supplement, especially if you are finding it difficult to eat properly.

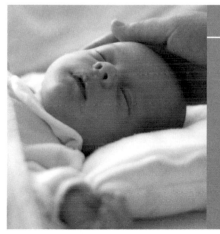

AROMATIC essential oils can be used to improve the quality of your own sleep

• Consult a homœopath for professional advice for treating your baby's insomnia.

• Explore acupuncture for yourself, to relieve stress associated with insomnia. Your practitioner should be able to show you how to rub acupressure points on your baby to help him or her sleep too.

• Use relaxing essential oils such as lavender in your bath water.

• If you are up most of the night with your baby, employ help during the day so that you can catch up on your sleep then.

• Keep to a routine with your baby as far as possible – especially

around bedtime. Don't over-stimulate your baby before bed, and follow the same pattern every evening – bath, last feed, cuddle, and soft sleepy music.

• Learn baby massage (see page 79) which will help to soothe a restless infant.

• If you can't get time out for a nap, try at least to take 10 minutes alone to meditate. If you're stressed, your baby will be too. If you're calm, then your baby will be too.

• Reassure yourself. If you're not getting the sleep you need, the sleep you do get becomes more intense in order to compensate, according to research at the Edinburgh Sleep Centre. Your body makes deep restorative sleep a priority and puts it first in your sleep cycle. Even though you will still feel tired the next day, reminding yourself that your body is looking after itself is a good way to take the pressure off.

SAFETY FIRST

• Always lay babies on their back to go to sleep.
• Make sure their head is uncovered.
• Place their feet at the foot of the cot, with the bedclothes tucked in firmly, and no higher than the shoulders, so that they can't wriggle underneath.

• Don't sleep with your baby in a narrow bed or on a sofa.
• Babies shouldn't get too hot or cold – an ideal room temperature is 16–20°C (61–68°F). You can buy a room thermometer from www.FSID.org.uk to make sure the room is neither too hot or cold.

Connecting With Your Baby

Mother's Instinct

Settling into a routine with your new baby can be daunting when everyone and their aunt wants to tell you what you should be doing. There's a huge amount of conflicting child rearing advice out there – and, as a new mother, anxious to do your best, it is often difficult to know which way to turn. This is when, more than ever, you need to tune into your innate maternal instinct. Your second best baby care expert is within you – while your best expert is the baby, programmed to let you know his or her needs.

 How best to care for your baby is a hugely divisive issue, with extreme views being equally popular. At one end of the spectrum there's the severe 'only cuddle your baby at feed-times' philosophy. At the other is the continuum concept, which involves the baby being literally a babe in arms 24/7. It is easy to see which of these is more conducive to connecting with your baby.

The continuum method – which means the baby is always held by an adult or an older child – is based on the behaviour of the Yequana tribe of South American Indians, whose babies almost never cry or vomit (unless extremely ill), and even grow into toddlers who are able to handle sharp tools like knives without hurting themselves because they have so closely and frequently observed how to use these safely.

With this method, babies sleep with their parents and are safe. However, despite the fact that one large study found that 50 per cent of UK babies are sleeping with their mothers at six months old, the advice of the Foundation for the Study of Infant Deaths is not to sleep with your baby – and always to settle him or her back in the crib if you sense that you are about to nod off. You may also feel that having to hold your baby all day long is too restrictive for you. But on the other hand, you need not feel guilty about picking your baby up if he or she cries. The sound of your heartbeat as you hold your baby is as comforting now as it was when he or she was still in the womb.

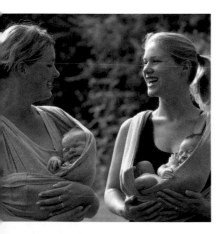

CONSTANT CONTACT suits some mothers and babies, but not all

READ UP

Baby care books serve a useful purpose, by suggesting different philosophies and approaches to child rearing. Read widely to get a sense of what feels right for you and your child; and use the books sensibly – don't let them bully you into regimes that feel uncomfortable.

Baby massage

Touch is hugely important to babies – in one study premature babies who had been stroked for 20 minutes a day for three weeks were better than a control group at intelligence tests, reading and comprehension when tested at the age of seven. They were also healthier – and it's thought that stroking increases levels of endorphins, which has a knock-on effect on the immune system.

A practitioner can show you how to massage your baby, and this will make you feel more confident about doing it alone. But if you have no qualms about getting started, here are a few pointers:

• Keep the room nice and warm, with soft music in the background.
• Place your baby on a soft, warm towel.
• Keep maintaining eye contact as much as possible.
• Use a simple vegetable oil such as almond or olive oil on a young baby.
• Start with your baby on his or her back. Warm a few drops of oil in your hands and start at the head, applying butterfly-light effleurage (superficial stroking) strokes from the back of the head to the front, using each hand in turn. Gradually move your hands outwards to take in the sides of the head, and the ears and neck, then lengthen the strokes more so you take in the chest, and then the tummy. Gently stroking the abdomen in a circular motion is very helpful if the baby is windy as it helps digestion.

VEGETABLE-BASED OIL such as olive oil is safe to use and gentle for your baby's skin

• Next clasp the arms and legs in turn, gently separating the toes and fingers and squeezing them very lightly while you continue to engage your baby with eye contact, singing or chatter.
• Finish by placing the baby on his or her front and using the same soft effleurage strokes from the shoulder blades to the buttocks, with small circular movements along the length of the back.

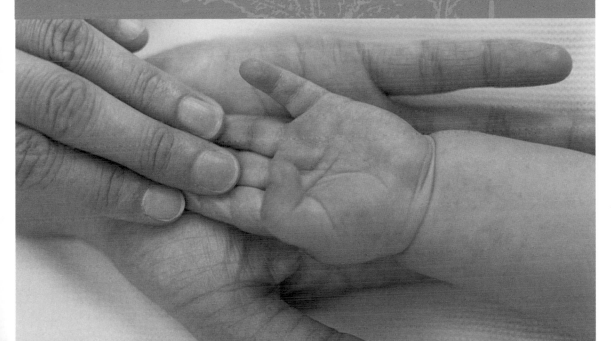

Natural Baby Care

Think Before You Buy

Your baby's skin is a living part of him or her, and it is the body's largest organ – so what you put on it matters enormously. If you use products containing synthetic ingredients, these chemicals risk irritating the skin on the outside and, over time, contributing to the cumulative build up of chemicals in his or her system, as it's hard for the body to get rid of them. Shop carefully when buying baby care products, and remember there is no legal definition for the word 'natural' – so when you see it on a product, you still need to do your detective work and read the label very carefully.

Start reading the labels of personal care products the way you do those of foods, and you may be shocked by what you discover. What may first read like gobbledegook if you're no science boffin could look like a cocktail of poisons once you've had a quick read of the 'what to avoid' section on the facing page. And, if you thought you were safe to stick to products aimed at babies, and made by household names, you were sadly mistaken. Shop shelves are bulging with baby care products containing chemicals that can irritate skin and eyes, along with some that have even been linked to cancer.

Pictures of babies covered in bubbles look really cute, but ask yourself: what is the magic ingredient that's making those bubbles? If – as is often the case – it is sodium lauryl sulphate (SLS), you may want to rethink what constitutes a happy bath time.

THINK CAREFULLY about the products you apply to your baby's skin

WHAT YOU MAY NEED

- Mild baby soap for washing, such as Organic Baby Soap from Neal's Yard Remedies. This is made with soothing calendula and is gentle and fine for baby skin, which is not oily and does not require strong products to clean it.
- Baby Barrier cream to prevent nappy rash.
- Baby bath-shampoo for gentle cleaning.
- An organic baby massage oil or baby oil – for massage and to gently remove cradle cap (dry flaky skin on the scalp).

What should I choose?

WHAT TO LOOK FOR

To moisturise the skin of a newborn baby, use only the simplest products, such as organic almond or sunflower oil, which you would consider good enough to eat. From about three months, you may like to introduce a mild baby soap or shampoo.

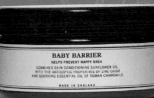

USE a quality barrier cream or shea butter to avoid skin irritation

BABY BARRIER
HELPS PREVENT NAPPY RASH
COMBINES SKIN CONDITIONING SUNFLOWER OIL
WITH THE ANTISEPTIC PROPERTIES OF ZINC OXIDE
AND SOOTHING ESSENTIAL OIL OF ROMAN CHAMOMILE.
MADE IN ENGLAND

ORGANIC
Your baby can absorb up to 90 per cent of what you put onto his or her skin, so by choosing organic skin care you can avoid the toxic cocktail of fertiliser and pesticide residues as well as many of the worst synthetic chemicals, which are banned from certified organic products.

ESSENTIAL OILS
There are a few very mild essential oils, such as lavender and Roman chamomile, that may be used on babies over three months old when properly diluted in a base oil, or in a carefully formulated baby product. However, don't use essential oils on a newborn baby and if any irritation or rashes develop, stop using anything you think might be causing it.

WHAT TO AVOID

DEA (DIETHANOLAMINE), MEA (MONETHANOLAMINE), TEA (TRIETHANOLAMINE)
These are ammonia derivatives used in foaming products (such as bubble bath and shampoo). They are potentially toxic and can irritate the skin, eyes and respiratory tract.

BENZOPHENONE-3, 4-METHYLBENZIDENE, CAMPHOR (4 MBC), HOMOSLATE, OCTYLDIMETHYL-PABA
Found in sunscreens and other cosmetics, these have estrogenic qualities and can proliferate cancer cells in breast and ovarian cancer.

PETROLATUM OR PARAFINNUM LIQUIDUM
These mineral oils are found in some baby oil; they can make skin more photosensitive and prone to sun damage, and will also block the pores of your baby's delicate skin.

PARABENS
These are preservatives that are found in many cosmetics and even foods and medicines for babies. They are oestrogen donors so may disrupt the delicate hormone balance, and some have been linked with breast tumours.

SODIUM LAURYL SULPHATE (SLS)
Found in baby bubble baths and other products, this is a harsh eye irritant that can cause permanent damage. In clinical studies on young animals, it has been shown that SLS is absorbed through the skin and then builds up in the eyes.

* These are a few examples provided by Foresight; for further information on toxic chemicals hidden in toiletries, go to www.foresight-preconception.org.uk

Nappies

Going Green

Nappies are a big issue for eco-conscious mothers. In a year, disposables make up about 2.6 per cent of the average household refuse – that is the equivalent in weight of nearly 70,000 double-decker buses, and these buses lined end-to-end would reach from London to Edinburgh. Opting for reusable cloth nappies reduces both the amount of waste sent for incineration and the amount of energy and non-renewable resources used to produce disposables. But how well will they fit in with your day-to-day life?

 Today's real nappies are worth looking into. They consist of a soft, absorbent nappy, with a separate disposable liner and an outer wrap that manages to be both waterproof and breathable. New designs fit snugly and safety pins have been replaced with Velcro fastenings, poppers and plastic grips for quick and easy fastening. There are over 30 different types and patterns, and they wash and dry easily.

The cost works out at about half that of the 4,000–6,000 disposables your baby would get through from birth to two-and-a-half, if you do your own laundering (the alternative is to use a laundry service), and you can reduce the environmental impact further by:

• Washing nappies at 60°C, and wraps at 40–60°C. You do not need to boil them.
• Using A-rated appliances to reduce energy and water consumption.
• Limiting the amount you use the tumble dryer, by drying them on a line or airer.
• Not using fabric conditioner, which will actually reduce absorbency.
• Using eco-friendly and bleach-free washing products.
• Using the same nappies for subsequent babies.

Test real nappies before making an investment, by using a loan service. For more information, go to www.realnappycampaign.com. If you do need to use disposables sometimes, there are biodegradable brands made from recycled fibres available nowadays.

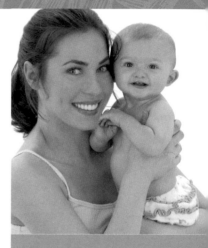

USE QUALITY PRODUCTS on your baby's skin to avoid irritation

NEED TO KNOW...

• Do your research in advance – ask other mums what they use, and look at any sample nappies you can get your hands on.
• Will real nappies fit in with your lifestyle? If you're organised about laundering, they may make life easier as you won't have to buy weekly supplies.

Nappy rash

Nappy rash happens to most babies at some point, and some seem to be particularly susceptible to it. Normally nappy rash will clear up in just a few days, but if you're at all concerned, consult your doctor. Using a baby balm or simple zinc and castor oil cream at each nappy change for a few days will usually sort out the problem; if not, then consulting a qualified homœopath may be worthwhile. Major causes include:

- Not changing your baby often enough – a nappy should be changed as soon as it's wet or soiled.
- Allergy to a washing powder or baby products (wipes can be full of chemicals, which may irritate your baby's skin); or sensitivity to lanolin (if you're using a wool wrap) or polyester (if you're using fleece liners).
- A change in food (usually temporary), once your baby is on solids.
- Your washing machine not cleaning your nappies thoroughly enough, leaving bacteria in the nappies, particularly if you wash at 40°C or below. Try washing at 60°C instead, with 5–10 drops of lavender or tea tree oil.

- Switching from disposable to cloth nappies – you may find there are a few days when your baby gets sore skin. This is simply just the change of environment and usually sorts itself out quickly.
- A rash that's red and flushed, sometimes with small pimples, is contact dermatitis, caused by bacteria creating ammonia, which burns the skin. This is classic 'nappy rash' and you can help your baby by changing the nappy more often, using a silk nappy liner, and using a different laundry detergent (choose one recommended for sensitive skins). Leave your baby's nappy off as much as possible to allow the skin to dry, and use a good quality cream to soothe the skin and act as a barrier. Left

untreated, the rash can lead to nastier infections.
- A bumpy sore rash that looks blistered or flaky, and much nastier than the nappy rash above, can arise if your baby is taking antibiotics as these disrupt the natural balance of good and bad bacteria in the gut, leading to a fungal infection. As well as the steps above, your baby will need a course of probiotics suitable for infants to help rebalance the gut flora.
- A dry, scaly or flaky rash that extends outside the nappy area is likely to be eczema. This can be brought on by sensitivity to products or detergent, so only use simple, natural, skin-friendly products. If the eczema seems to persist, take your baby to see a homœopath.

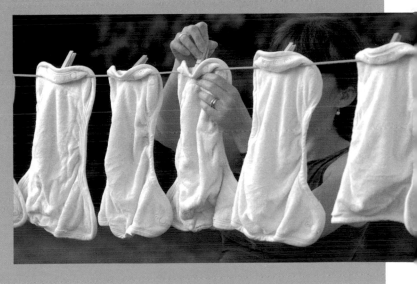

Baby Health

Natural Healing

If you plan to bring your baby up holistically, and have already established a rapport with a practitioner during pregnancy, take your healthy baby along in the first six weeks for a discussion about the way forward with his or her health care. Such a visit will inspire and encourage you, so you can move on with confidence. Knowledge is power, but use it wisely. There will be times when home remedies are all that you need – but others when expert advice is crucial.

 To treat simple things, there are a number of self-help remedies that you can try at home, but there are other times when you will need to take your baby along for some expert help from a qualified practitioner.

Cranial osteopathy

Cranial osteopathy is useful for a baby who is sleeping badly following birth trauma (see pages 76–7), and for babies who were delivered with forceps or ventouse, or who have colic.

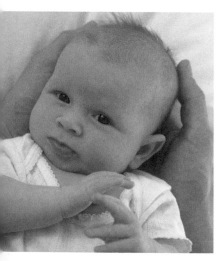

CRANIAL OSTEOPATHY benefits many newborns

Herbalism

Herbalism provides help for:
• Colic – try a weak infusion of fennel or dill three or four times a day, or drink a cupful yourself before breastfeeding.
• Coughs – for very young babies, add a few drops of eucalyptus or pine oil to a bowl of hot water and place it beside the baby; for babies over six months, add two drops of each essential oil to a little vegetable oil and massage onto the chest to help loosen phlegm.
• Conjunctivitis – bathe the eye with a few drops of breast milk or an infusion of marigold, which has good antiseptic properties.
• Eczema or rashes – apply marigold ointment three times a day or apply mashed warm cabbage leaves to the skin to soothe inflammation).

Homœopathy

Homœopathy can help earache. Try Aconite 30c for babies in severe pain or who have been out in cold air, Belladonna 30c if flushed, or Chamomilla 30c if they are restless

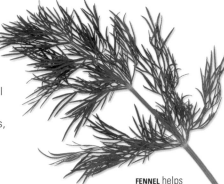

FENNEL helps ease colic

FLOWER REMEDIES

Simple and safe, flower remedies are great for babies and dosage is the same as for adults.

Try the following:
• White chestnut if your baby can't sleep.
• Mimulus for an anxious baby.
• Rescue remedy – an all rounder worth having in your baby bag.

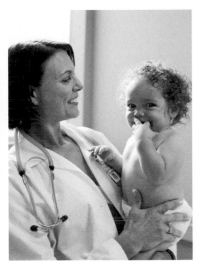

A HEALTHY BABY is a happy baby

and irritable. Give the remedy every eight hours for two days. For a teething baby, apply Chamomilla teething granules directly to the gums three or four times a day. For colic, try Colocynth 6c or Magnesium phosphoricum 6c four times a day during the attack.

The immunisation debate

All infants are offered a series of immunisations usually starting with diphtheria, tetanus, polio and Hib at two months. Some parents choose to delay certain vaccinations until their baby's immune system is more developed, or even decline them altogether. The controversy about the Measles, Mumps and Rubella (MMR) immunisation is well explained in the booklet *Understanding MMR* by Lara Sussman, available from Neal's Yard Remedies.

If you want more information about the pros and cons of vaccination in general contact the Informed Parent for their newsletter (www.informedparent.org).

What's wrong?

DIARRHOEA AND VOMITING – are signs of gastroenteritis, and babies can deteriorate rapidly as they are quick to dehydrate. Ask your pharmacist for rehydration salts to replace the lost minerals quickly, and seek medical advice about what to give your baby to eat if he or she is on solids.

FEVER – a baby temperature over 38°C is a fever, and a reaction to illness. It's the body's way of fighting an infection, as the bugs causing it cannot live much above normal body temperature. Seek medical advice for any baby under a year who has a fever (and urgently when the baby is under six weeks), and try to get your baby's temperature down by cooling. Take any clothes off but leave the nappy on. Cover him or her in bed with a sheet but not blankets. Give plenty of cold drinks. Use a fan to cool the room, and wipe the forehead with a tepid flannel. The homœopathic combination remedy Aconite, Belladonna and Chamomilla 30c can be given every two hours to help reduce the fever.

RASHES – check out any rash, especially if accompanied by any form of malaise. A septicaemic rash

(accompanying meningitis) will only appear as a late symptom – and it's a rash that doesn't go away when a tumbler is pressed to it – but beware first of other symptoms such as pallor, fever and vomiting, a stiff neck, high pitched crying, and dislike of bright light. Seek urgent medical advice when any combination of these symptoms occurs. Chicken pox and measles (on the rise again) also cause a rash and the latter is a notifiable disease. If your health practice has a leaflet on baby rashes, grab a copy and keep it in your medical box for speedy reference.

Other signs your baby is generally unwell include:
• A usually active child moping and becoming uninterested in her toys.
• A child who previously slept and ate well but is now constantly irritable.
• Constant crying.
• Dry nappies for more than nine to 12 hours.

CAMOMILE INFUSION can be given to children to help reduce a fever

Baby Blues

Feeling Low

When we talk of the baby blues, we're referring to the emotional turbulence that about half of all new mothers experience shortly after birth, and around the time that their milk comes in. The symptoms – feeling very emotional and upset – may last for a few hours or, at most, a few days, and then they disappear. But if your blues seem to go on for longer, don't delay talking to someone who can help you.

 Mild post-natal blues can be treated with a herbal tonic of balm, borage, skullcap and oats to balance the hormones and nervous system. Make a decoction to drink three times a day, or take the herbs in tincture form. Essential oils can also lift your mood – choose any one or two of geranium, neroli or rose, and add a couple of drops diluted in base oil to your bath water, or use them in a vegetable oil for massage.

But if you carry on feeling low for longer than a few days, do talk to your doctor or natural therapist urgently, because post-natal depression can become a serious and ongoing problem if it's not dealt with properly in its early stages. Sadly, as figures for the number of sufferers are vague, it seems that too few women report their symptoms or seek help, often seeing it as a sign of weakness or failure on their part. This is a great shame, because we all know that depression is the common cold of mental health, affecting one in four of us at some point in our lives, and developing just as randomly as any commonplace physical health problem. Yet the statistics for the numbers of women with post-natal illness (or post-natal depression) are woolly – ranging from one in ten to one in five of new mothers. Equally shameful is the fact that little information about the condition is given to expectant mothers – which must only serve to fuel the stigma that surrounds it.

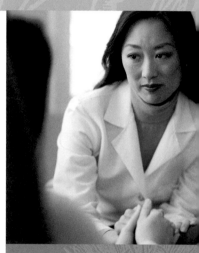

FLOWER OILS can lift your mood

TIRED ALL THE TIME

• Talk to your midwife or health visitor about your emotions – they are as important as your physical health, and nothing to be embarrassed about.

• A professional should be on the look-out for signs of post-natal depression, and should be able to offer good advice.

Knowing the signs

If your baby blues seem to be getting worse rather than better, and the symptoms are becoming more distressing, depression could be developing – although for some women the baby blues pass and then, several weeks after the birth, depression starts to set in. You may not even recognise what is happening because, since the baby's arrival, everything has changed – and it is easy to simply blame your symptoms on all the new demands. If you are looking after yourself properly, you have to ask yourself why you are not coping. And this may be due to some degree of depression – or post-natal illness – if you notice several of the following symptoms:

• You feel permanently tired and lethargic.
• Simple household chores seem too much effort.
• You can't be bothered to bathe, dress properly or care for your appearance.
• You suffer from head, neck or back pain.
• You feel generally unwell.
• You are anxious – worrying unjustifiably about the baby and other members of the family.
• You can't cope with meeting friends or answering the door.
• You experience confusion or panic in an everyday situation.
• You can't relax, no matter how much you know you should.
• You develop obsessional thoughts.

• You can't concentrate on books, television programmes or even conversation.
• You sleep badly.

If you go to your doctor you may be offered tranquillisers or antidepressants, with the aim of 'buying time' for your recovery. However, the risk of being offered drugs you do not want should not deter you from talking to your doctor. Many practices have counsellors attached to them, and you may get some talk therapy on the NHS. Your doctor should also know of support groups or specialist therapy in your area. Aromatherapy, homœopathy, herbalism and acupuncture can all help to treat the symptoms of post-natal depression, so consider visiting a qualified practitioner.

It is also important to take a good multivitamin and mineral supplement, as a shortage of essential nutrients such as zinc can add to the symptoms of depression. During your recovery you can help yourself a lot by believing in your ability to get better. But you need patience and you have to understand that recovery will probably take time.

Take as much rest as you can – tiredness makes depression worse – and try to rest on your bed (sleeping if possible) every day. Avoid late nights and try to get someone else to feed or look after the baby for a couple of hours.

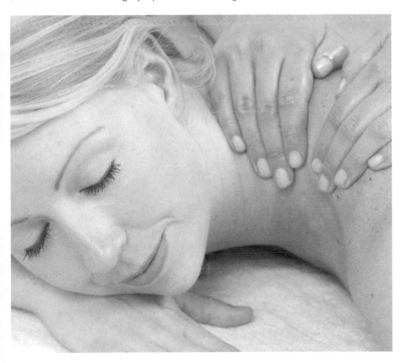

AROMATHERAPY MASSAGE can help boost your mood

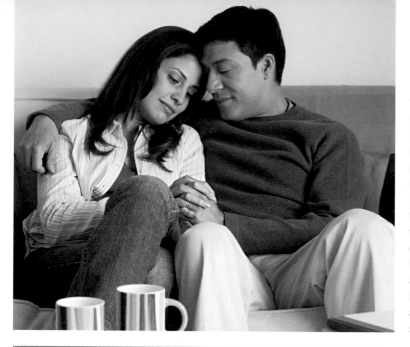

Try not to go without food for long periods, as hypoglycaemia – low blood sugar – can make things much worse for you. It's also a good idea to find small chores you can easily complete as these will help occupy you, once you're ready for them. Being just busy enough will take away those feelings of uselessness that come with having nothing to do when you are depressed. This is sometimes known as 'polish your shoes' advice, but – done slowly and steadily – simple tasks can help.

BEATING THE BLUES

If you're looking for some independent help, the following are all worth considering:

- Cranial osteopathy – cranial osteopaths believe that post-natal depression can be caused by the downward displacement of the uterus following birth and the resultant tug on the pituitary gland via the dura (this is a continuous thin membrane that lines the brain and spinal cord). Some cranial osteopaths claim they can relieve post-natal depression in just two weeks.

- Acupuncture – this has a good record for treating depression of all types.

- Homœopathy – being treated homœopathically throughout pregnancy may prevent post-natal depression. Also, if it does develop, there are some useful homœopathic remedies that an experienced homœopath would be able to prescribe.

- Herbalism – tinctures of St John's Wort, chaste berry (agnus castus), borage and oats, used in equal parts and taken in a 5 ml dose three times a day, can help. Borage (starflower) oil is specifically recommended for post-natal depression

FLOWER POWER – find natural cures for the blues

and can be taken in 500 mg capsules three to four times a day in addition to your post-natal formula.

- The essential oils of jasmine, clary sage and ylang-ylang are also recommended for post-natal depression. Mix one drop of each to 10 ml of base oil then add one drop to your bath water, or evaporate one drop in an essential oil burner.

You're not alone

Talking through your problems with someone who's been through the same thing can also be enormously helpful, so do seek out local support groups, or web groups. This is particularly helpful if, every time you go to a mother and baby gathering, you come away feeling as if everyone else is having a better time of it than you. Many, many women do not take to motherhood straight away, and this is entirely normal – a lot of routine baby care is drudgery, and it's hardly surprising if you do not feel on cloud nine all the time, especially if you're used to being very independent. You just need to find some kindred spirits who feel the same way – and to remember you can still love your baby and be a good mother while also feeling bored and frustrated by some aspects of your role.

HEALTHY MIND

• Seek out kindred spirits.

• Keep a structure to your day – but don't become a slave to routine, or you risk being stressed if things go wrong.

• Always find something to look forward to.

KEEP YOUR OXYGEN MASK ON

Remember the lovely analogy with using your oxygen mask before helping someone else with theirs? It was given to me by a wonderful life coach, Annabel Sutton, author of the Neal's Yard Remedies book "52 Ways to Handle It", and is worth remembering here because, even if you seem to have got through the post-natal period without any emotional turbulence (problems are not obligatory!), none of us should take our happiness for granted. Work at it by treating yourself to facials and massages. A study in Nature Neuroscience found that tender stroking triggers activity in the area of the brain that controls emotional health. Your body has been through a lot with pregnancy, birth and now breastfeeding, so don't try to be the do-it-all hero – book yourself time off and enjoy it. The following tips should also help you to hang on to happiness on the days when this seems tough:

• Hang out with cheerful people. Joy is catching and in one study scientists asked volunteers to scowl at happy faces – but the volunteers found it hard to stop their own mouths from curling upwards!

• Try to be upbeat. Start by giving yourself positive little messages, such as 'I can handle this!' – and never say anything more critical to yourself than you would to a colleague you respect.

• Sleep yourself happy – sleep rejuvenates the brain's cerebral cortex, which drives moods, decision making and short-term memory. If you stint on it, your mood will plummet.

• Be thankful. In studies, people who strongly agree with statements such as 'I have so much to be thankful for' are less depressed than their ungrateful counterparts. Get in practice by taking a few minutes a day to reflect on at least five things you appreciate.

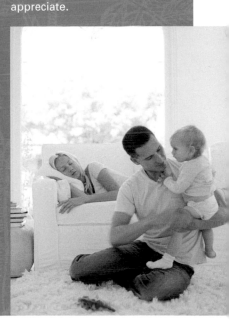

Keep Up The Good Work!

Putting It All Together

This book has been your companion for a few months now – seeing you through from early pregnancy to the first few weeks of your baby's life. If it has introduced you to new ideas about health and the environment, there will probably be only one way forward for you now – we all want our children to have the best chances in life – and we hope we have given you something that you can carry with you as your family grows.

If you didn't know it before, you now know the importance of:

A healthy diet

You ate well to create the right conditions for conception and a healthy baby, and you now know the importance of food for your own mental as well as physical health. The better your diet, the better your child's will be, too. Keep up the good work with a fresh and varied diet. Make your five-a-day the minimum, not the maximum, number of fruit and vegetables you eat; include oily fish in your diet at least once a week, and make the most of foods that are seasonal and locally grown. If you don't already use a fruit and vegetable box scheme, look into those that are delivered in your area. They're an opportunity to eat organically, and inevitably open your mind to new foods that might not make it onto your usual menu.

A chemical-free life

The chemicals you've been exposed to can affect your fertility, and the health of your growing baby. They can cause allergies, and may build up a toxic load that increases your risk of cancer. Go chemical-free as much as you can, by carefully reading the labels on household products, cosmetics and toiletries, and eating organically as far as possible. A good diet with the right balance of minerals will help you to flush toxins from chemical build-up out of your system.

A good exercise routine

If you were a regular exerciser before your pregnancy, you will have been able to adapt almost

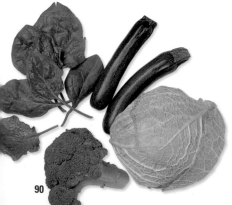

A VEGETABLE BOX scheme is a good way of getting quality seasonal produce

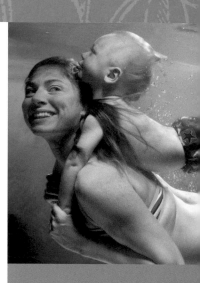

NATURAL MOTHER

Being a natural mum is as much about having confidence in your own instinct as it is about giving your family a healthy diet, and knowing where to find holistic remedies when they're needed. Enjoy your new role, and learn from all it has to offer you.

anything you normally do while you were expecting. If you weren't, you will still have been able to take some gentle exercise – even if it was just a daily walk. Now build on that and walk further and faster. Walking with a buggy is a great way to get fit, and studies prove that the children of mothers who exercise regularly are more likely to be active and sporty than the children of inactive mums. In an era when childhood obesity is becoming an epidemic, and we have the first ever generation of children who are expected to die before their parents, what better reason is there to get moving?

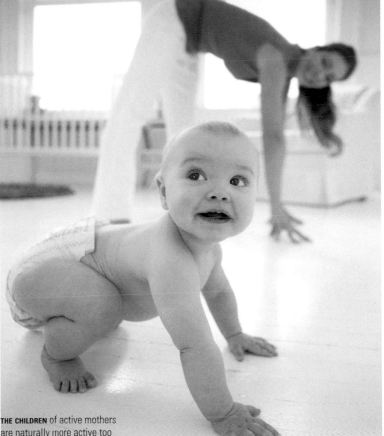

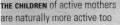
THE CHILDREN of active mothers are naturally more active too

Rest and relaxation

Even if you were a yoga and meditation virgin before pregnancy, our simple exercises may have given you a taste for both. They are great ways to calm and restore the body, and it's well worth remembering that the word 'meditation' comes from the same Latin root medicus as medicine and medicate – meaning 'to cure'. The health benefits are numerous, but to make the most of them you need to build up to sitting for 20 minutes in stillness. Practise with a group or teacher until you feel confident doing it yourself.

Home remedies

This book is peppered with lots of remedies you can make for yourself at home, using herbs, tinctures and flower remedies. Keeping a supply of these at home, for common complaints, is empowering and enables you to take control of your own small health problems when you need to.

Holistic medicine

If pregnancy was the catalyst that introduced you to holistic, complementary medicine, use it now to keep your good health. It can help to relieve chronic conditions and prevent others by working on the body as a whole and not simply waiting for symptoms of ill health to arise. Building up a relationship with a few practitioners that you really trust   for you and your baby – can stand you in good stead for years to come. Especially useful at this time, for both you and your growing family, are an experienced homœopath and cranial osteopath.

Hanging on to happiness

Be happy with the person you are and don't set too high standards for yourself. Health and happiness really do go together, and being content with being so so is great for anyone's self-esteem. If you get upset when things aren't perfect, you will know too well how stressful perfectionism and lofty aspirations can be. Make it your happiness rule that you will never be a competitive mum, just the natural mother you are.

Index

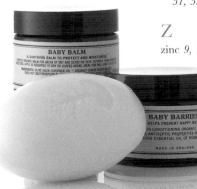

Neal's Yard Remedies

Practising What We Preach

Neal's Yard Remedies was born in 1981. We like to think of ourselves as pioneers. Today, awareness and interest in natural remedies, skin and body care are on the increase. But when we opened our first shop in Covent Garden, we were one of the few pushing against the synthetic chemical approach to skin and health care that had been adopted by much of the industry. Our vision was to bring the expertise of the apothecary and a holistic approach to health and beauty to local people and their communities.

 What matters to us are people, their health and their happiness. We're obsessed with discovering and delivering natural ways to improve health and well-being and delivering outstanding natural and organic skin- and body-care products. We also believe passionately that our environment is of vital importance, both in its own right, and as the source of many of the plants and herbs vital to our well-being. That's why we actively support and promote organic farming and the use of certified organic ingredients in our products.

We encourage you to take responsibility for your own health. We do so by offering a wide range of products, providing therapy rooms where you can experience a variety of natural therapies, and teaching courses in natural medicine. We aim to make natural medicine accessible to everyone. We do this by supplying high-quality natural remedies at a fair price and by educating people on their safe and effective use. Ill health gives us the opportunity to learn something about ourselves, and creating health is only possible when we actively participate in that learning experience. Using natural remedies may assist us in the transformative process of becoming healthier.

Are our products really safer?

Our commitment to using safe, natural ingredients with a recognized therapeutic tradition creates products that are beneficial to both you and the environment. All our products undergo strict testing to ensure they're safe and effective to use.

WHAT DOES ORGANIC MEAN?

Respecting nature. No pesticides. No genetic modification. Local production wherever we can. It also means honesty and integrity. No false claims. That's why Neal's Yard Remedies follow the strict standards set by the Soil Association, and why we put their symbol on our organic products.

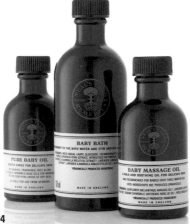

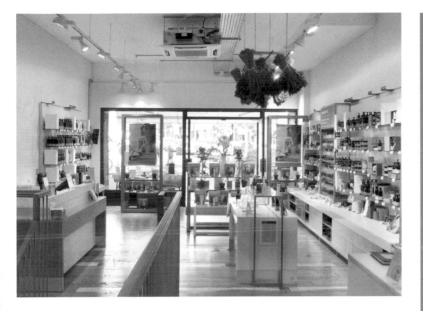

OUR COMMITMENT TO YOU

We always aim to make our products as effective and as natural as possible. We hand-make them ourselves from ingredients with proven properties.

WE USE
Organic ingredients
Vibrant plant extracts
Plant-based ingredients
Pure essential oils
Therapeutic extracts

NO genetically modified materials
NO artificial colours
NO petrochemicals
NO synthetic fragrances
NO parabens or sodium lauryl sulphate

Mail order
Tel: 0845 262 3145
E-mail: mailorder@nealsyardremedies.com
Address: Mail Order
Peacemarsh
Gillingham
Dorset
SP8 4EU

Customer service advice line
Trained staff on the advice line can give advice and information on products and remedies, help you find a local practitioner, as well as help you with complaints or feedback about a product or service.
Tel: 01747 834 634
E-mail: advice@nealsyardremedies.com
Opening times: Monday–Friday 9am–5.30pm

Shops & Therapy Rooms
We have shops and therapy rooms throughout the UK. To find your nearest one, check out our website or phone Customer Services on 01747 834 634

Website
You can purchase all of our products from our website, which we hope you will also find a mine of information.
www.nealsyardremedies.com

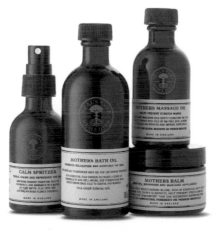

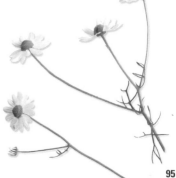

Further resources and reading

Resources

ACTIVE BIRTH CENTRE
Tel: 02072 816760
Web: www.activebirthcentre.com

FORESIGHT ASSOCIATION
Tel: 01243 868001
Web: www.foresight-preconception.org.uk

GENERAL COUNCIL AND REGISTER OF NATUROPATHS
Tel: 08707 456984
Web: www.naturopathy.org.uk

INTERNATIONAL ASSOCIATION OF INFANT MASSAGE (IAIM)
Tel: 02089 899597
Web: www.iaim.org.uk

INTERNATIONAL FEDERATION OF PROFESSIONAL AROMATHERAPISTS
Tel: 01455 637987
Web: www.ifparoma.org

LA LECHE LEAGUE
Tel: 0845 120 2918
Web: www.laleche.org.uk

NATIONAL INSTITUTE OF MEDICAL HERBALISTS (NIMH)
Tel: 01392 426022
Web: www.nimh.org.uk

THE INFORMED PARENT
Tel: 01903 212969
Web: www.informedparent.co.uk

THE REAL NAPPY CAMPAIGN
Tel: 0845 850 0606
Web: www.realnappycampaign.com

THE SOCIETY OF HOMEOPATHS
Tel: 0845 450 6611
Web: www.homeopathy-soh.org

Reading

ALTERNATIVE MATERNITY, by Nicky Wesson (Vermilion)

ESSENTIAL OILS, by Susan Curtis (Haldane Mason)

HOLISTIC HERBAL, by David Hoffman (Healing Arts Press)

HOMOEOPATHY, by Rebecca Wells (Haldane Mason)

NATURAL HEALING FOR WOMEN, by Susan Curtis and Romy Fraser (Thorsons)

NEAL'S YARD NATURAL REMEDIES, by Curtis, Frase, Kohler (Winter Press)

THE ALTERNATIVE PREGNANCY HANDBOOK, by Dr Tanvir Jamil and Karen Evennett (Piatkus Books)

THE OPTIMUM NUTRITION BIBLE, by Patrick Holford (Piatkus Books)

WONDERFOODS, by Natalie Savona (Quadrille)

Karen Evennett graduated from University College London before training as a journalist and eventually choosing to speciali in writing about women's heal She has a special interest in holistic health, and is a prolific contributor to women's magaz and the author of 11 other women's health books includin *The Alternative Pregnancy Handbook* (Piatkus), which she co-wrote with Dr Tanvir Jamil.

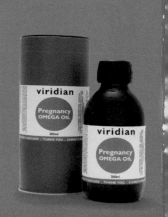

Viridian Nutrition was founded in 1999 on two fundamental principles – to produce an exceptional range of vitamins, minerals and herbs and to make a significant contribution to the funds of environmental, children's and other charities. Viridian has won numerous awards for the company's ethic and was named best buy in Ethical Consumer magazine's review of vitamins.

Viridian Nutrition
Tel: +44 (0)1327 878050
www.viridian-nutrition.com